Thyroid Health Cookbook

50+ Simple and Delicious Recipes That Will Boast Thyroid Health!

BY - Alain Duke

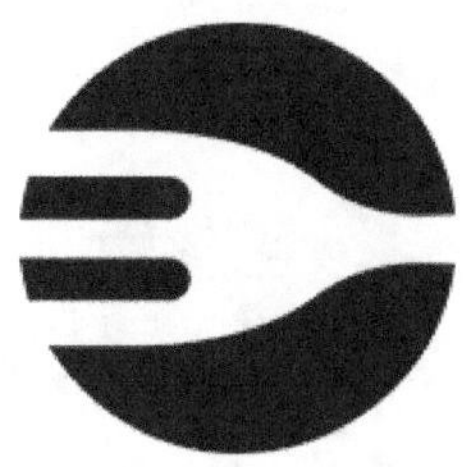

Copyright Notification

The content of this book cannot be sold, published, printed, copied, disseminated, or distributed without the permission of the author. If you possess an unauthorized copy, it is necessary to delete it right away and acquire the legal version.

It should be noted that the author does not accept any liability for the actions taken by the reader based on the information provided in the book. Although the author has made every effort to ensure the accuracy of the information, it is crucial to proceed with caution while implementing the content. The book is intended solely as an informational resource.

Table of Contents

Introduction

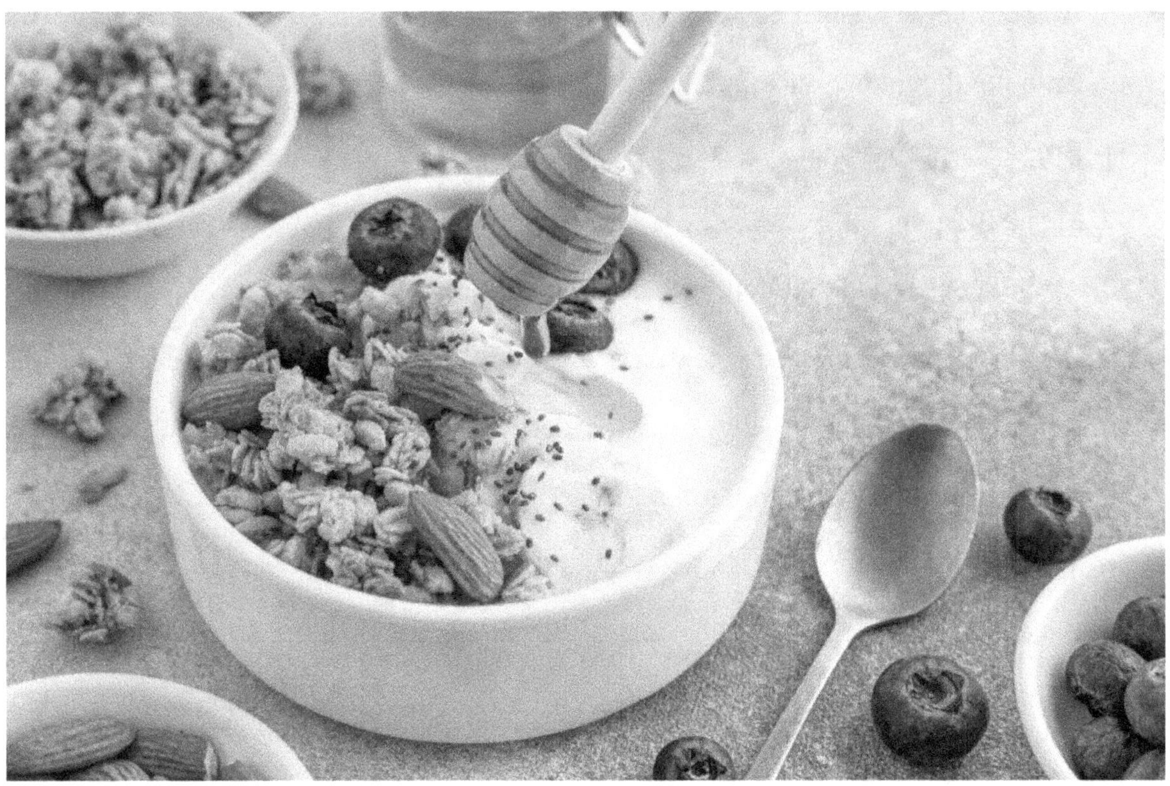

Are you tired of feeling sluggish, battling unexplained weight gain, and wrestling with persistent mood swings? Do you ever wonder why your energy levels seem to plummet, leaving you dragging yourself through the day? Have you ever felt the frustration of knowing something is not quite right with your body, but not knowing where to turn for answers? If any of these questions resonate with you, you're not alone. Millions of people around the world grapple with these issues daily, often without realizing that one tiny gland in their body, the thyroid, might hold the key to their well-being.

Thyroid problems can be a silent tormentor, affecting our lives in ways we might not even suspect. The thyroid, that unassuming butterfly-shaped gland in our neck, plays a pivotal role in regulating our metabolism, energy levels, and overall health. When it's not functioning optimally, it can wreak havoc on our bodies and minds. But the good news is that understanding your thyroid's needs and nurturing it through the right diet can bring about transformative changes in your life.

This Thyroid Health Cookbook is a culinary journey that will empower you to take control of your thyroid health and rediscover the vitality you deserve. In this book, we've meticulously crafted 50 delicious recipes, each accompanied by a mouthwatering image and a detailed description, to help you nourish your thyroid and reclaim your well-being.

So, if you're ready to embark on a journey to better thyroid health, if you're ready to bid farewell to exhaustion, weight struggles, and brain fog, and if you're ready to embrace a vibrant and energetic life, then this is the right book for you. Let's begin this transformative journey together, one delicious bite at a time. Your thyroid will thank you, and so will your body and soul. Welcome to the Thyroid Health Cookbook – your roadmap to a healthier you.

Chapter 1: Breakfast Recipes

1. Frozen Chocolate Milk

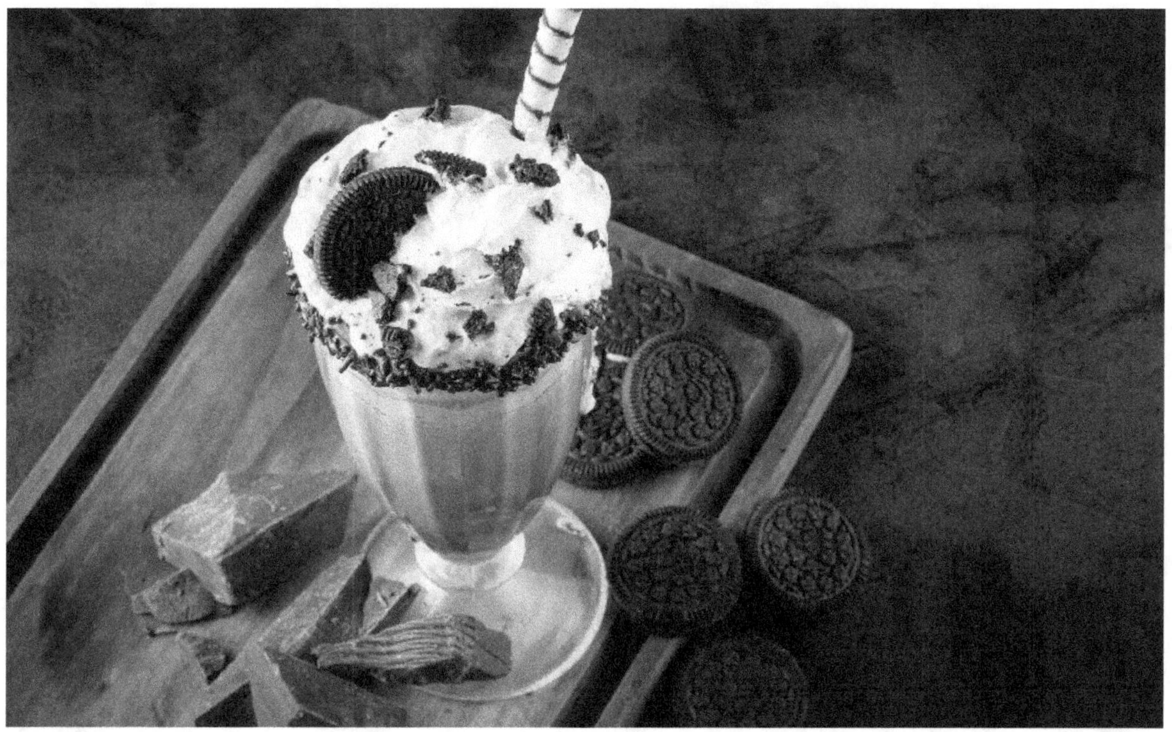

Cocoa powder is made from dried, roasted cacao beans, which are actually classified as seeds of the fruit of the Theobroma cacao tree. Cocoa powder is known for its high antioxidant content because of its abundance of polyphenolic flavonoids that can help reduce the risk of heart disease.

Cooking time: 0 minutes

Servings: 2

Ingredients:

- 2 frozen bananas
- 1½ cups unsweetened coconut milk beverage
- 2 teaspoons unsweetened cocoa powder

Instructions:

In a high-speed blender, combine the bananas, coconut milk, and cocoa powder.

Blend on high speed until completely smooth.

2. Grain-Free Cassava Pancakes

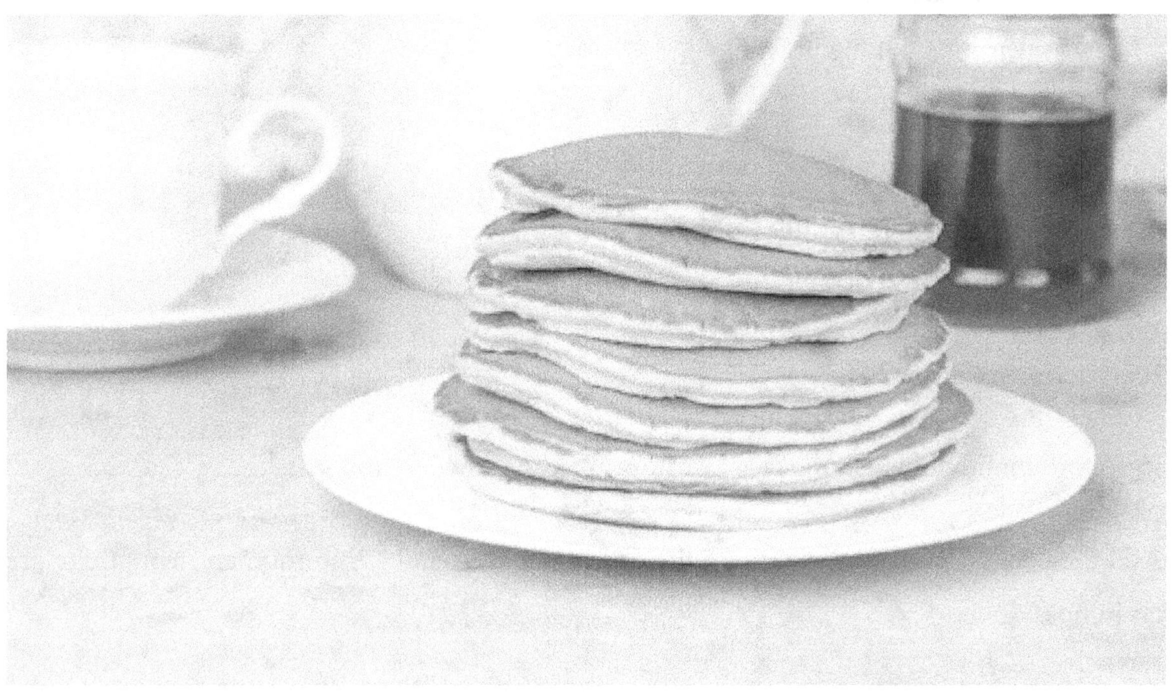

A weekend breakfast staple, many people miss pancakes on their elimination diet. These cassava pancakes are a great alternative to enjoy on occasion. They are denser than traditional pancakes and have a neutral flavor, making them perfect for both sweet and savory toppings.

Cooking time: 15 minutes

Servings: 4

Ingredients:

- 1¼ cups cassava flour
- ½ teaspoon baking powder
- ¼ teaspoon salt
- 1 cup unsweetened coconut milk beverage
- 1 teaspoon pure vanilla extract
- 2 tablespoons coconut oil

Instructions:

In a medium bowl, whisk the cassava flour, baking powder, and salt.

Add the coconut milk and vanilla to the dry ingredients and stir to mix, ensuring there are no lumps.

In a cast-iron skillet over medium heat, heat the coconut oil.

Once hot, add ¼-cup portions of batter to the pan. Cook for 2 minutes. Flip the pancakes and cook for 3 minutes more, or until cooked through. Repeat with the remaining batter.

3. Green Tea & Ginger Oatmeal

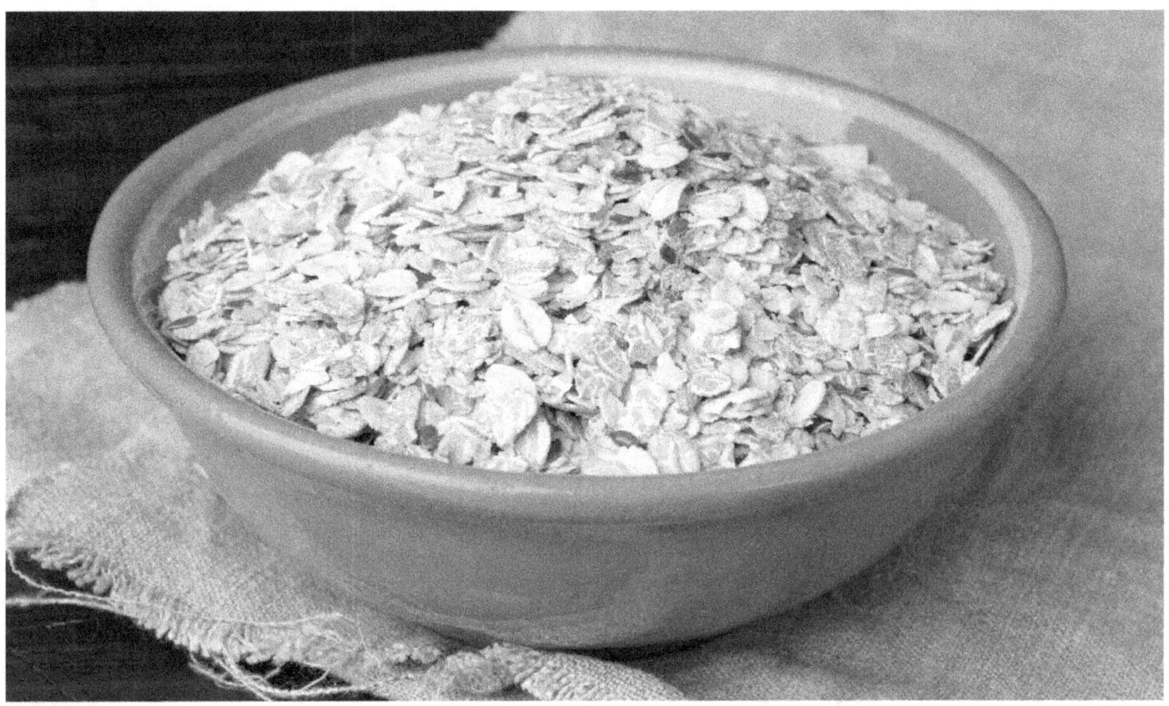

Enjoy the amazing health benefits of both green tea and ginger in one warm, comforting breakfast bowl. Green tea is a powerful beverage packed with antioxidants such as polyphenols and catechins that can help prevent cell damage.

Cooking time: 7 minutes

Servings: 4

Ingredients:

- 4 green tea bags
- 3¼ cups filtered water
- ¼ teaspoon salt
- 2 cups old-fashioned rolled oats
- 2 teaspoons grated peeled fresh ginger
- 2 teaspoons pure maple syrup
- 4 dried figs, sliced

Instructions:

In a medium saucepan over medium-high heat, combine the tea bags, water, and salt. Bring to a boil. Remove and discard the tea bags.

Stir in the oats. Reduce the heat to a simmer. Cook, uncovered, for 5 minutes, stirring occasionally.

Stir in the ginger and maple syrup. Cook for 2 minutes more. Remove from the heat and top with the figs (if using).

4. Sweet Potato Sausage Hash

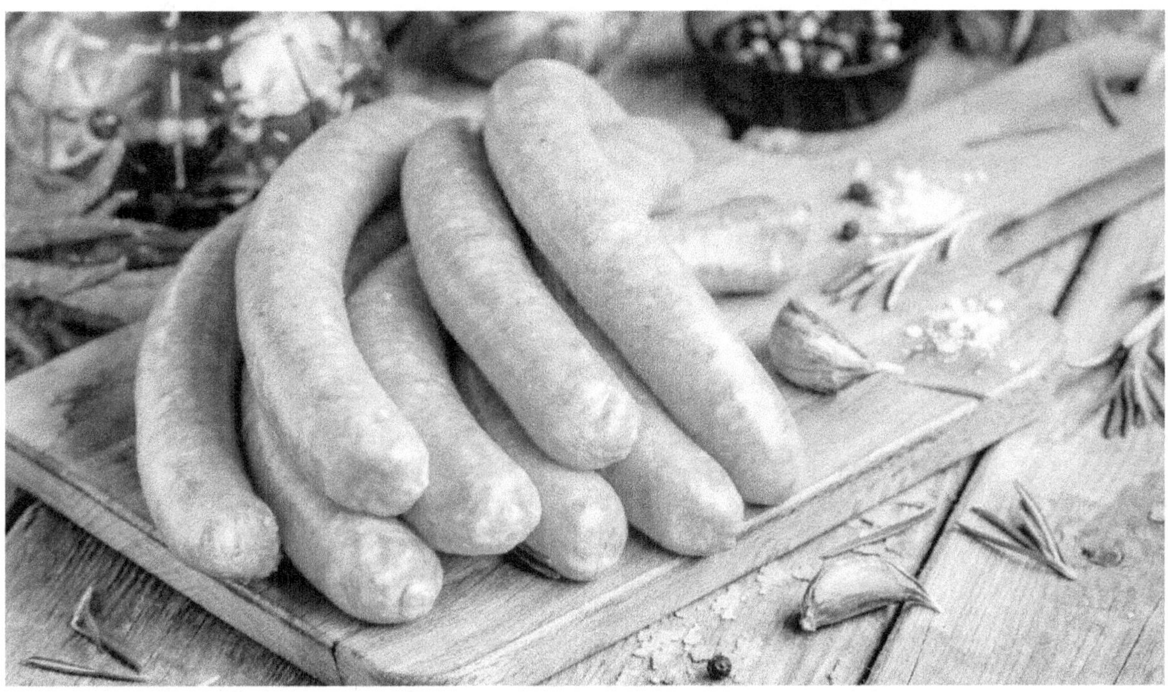

Hash is a classic dish made with chopped meat, potatoes, and spices that are mixed and cooked together. This version is prepared with ground pork, a high-quality protein source that includes many important nutrients such as iron, B vitamins, and dried herbs.

Cooking time: 26 minutes

Servings: 4

Ingredients:

- ¼ cup water
- 2 tablespoons pure maple syrup
- 2 tablespoons Brown Bacon "Butter"
- 1 cup finely chopped white onion
- 1-pound sweet potatoes, cut into ½-inch cubes
- 8 ounces ground breakfast sausage
- ¼ teaspoon salt

Instructions:

In a small bowl, whisk together the water and maple syrup. Set aside.

In a large cast-iron skillet, heat the bacon "butter" over medium heat and sauté the onions for 2 minutes, until they begin to turn translucent.

Add the sweet potatoes and salt and cook for 10 minutes, stirring frequently, until they are tender and slightly browned.

Using a spoon, move the onions and sweet potatoes to the outside of the pan.

Increase the heat to medium-high and add the sausage to the center of the pan. Allow to cook for 2 minutes. Constantly stir the sausage, allowing it to brown.

Stir the onion and sweet potatoes with the sausage until mixed well.

Using a spatula, flatten all the ingredients into a single layer and cook for 3 to 5 minutes without stirring, allowing the ingredients to brown.

Flip the ingredients and cook for 3 to 5 more minutes, until browned on the other side.

Add the water and maple syrup mixture to deglaze the pan, stirring well and scraping up any pieces left on the bottom of the pan.

Cook for 1 to 2 minutes, stirring well. Serve once all the water has evaporated.

5. Penne with Avocado

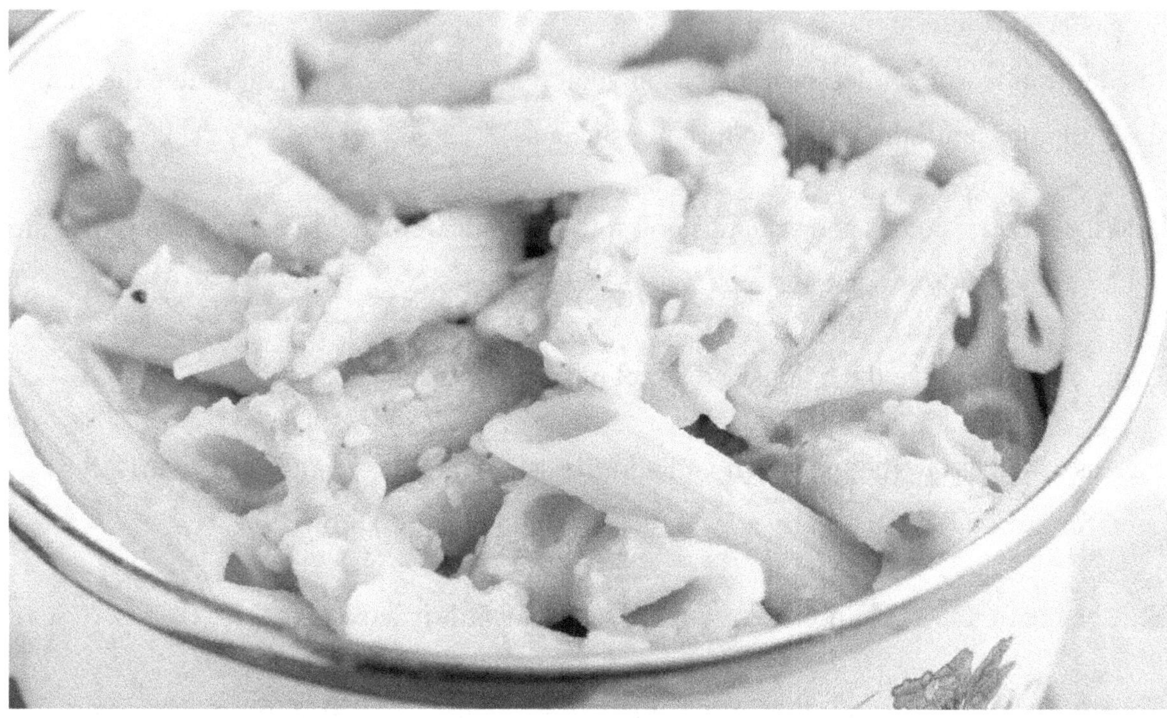

Packed with healthy fats, fiber, and vitamins, it's a nutritious delight. Avocado offers heart-healthy monounsaturated fats and potassium, while the pasta provides energizing carbs.

Cooking time: 30 minutes

Servings: 4

Ingredients:

- 4-oz penne
- 1 tsp olive oil
- 1 onion
- 1 pepper
- 1 garlic clove
- 1 tsp chili powder
- 1 tsp coriander
- ¼ tsp cumin seeds
- 1 lb. tomatoes
- 1 (10-oz) can sweetcorn
- 1 avocado
- ¼ lime

Instructions:

Cook the pasta for 10-15 minutes

In a pan, heat oil and sautéed onion, garlic and tomatoes.

Stir in water, corn and simmer for another 12-15 minutes.

Toss the avocado with lime juice.

Place the pasta in the pot, add remaining ingredients, and cook for another 2-3 minutes.

When ready, remove from heat and serve.

6. Cream of Cauliflower with Fruit

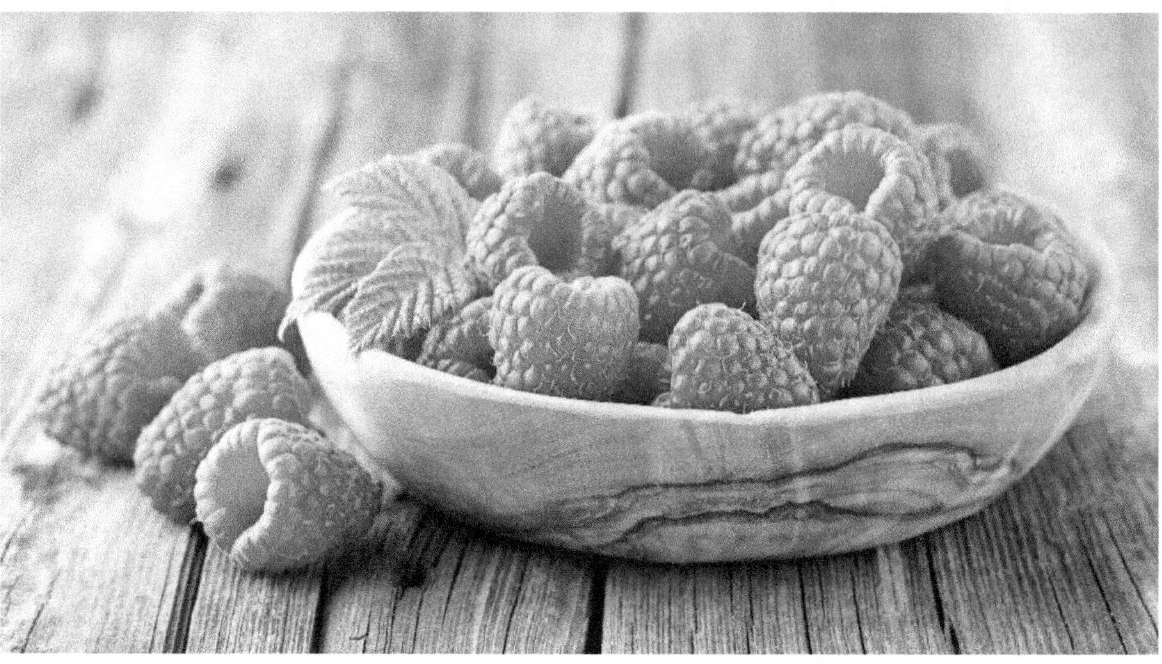

Breakfast can be hard for people adopting a Paleo or AIP diet because many traditional breakfast staples, such as oatmeal, are omitted. Thankfully, this recipe provides the same hearty, warming breakfast feeling without the grains or gluten. You can easily customize this sweet bowl like you would traditional oats.

Cooking time: 30 minutes

Servings: 4

Ingredients:

- 2 cups Creamy Cauliflower Grits
- ½ cup full-fat coconut milk
- 2 tablespoons pure maple syrup
- 2 tablespoons coconut flour
- 2 tablespoons unflavored collagen peptides (optional)
- ⅛ teaspoon pure vanilla extract
- 1/8 teaspoon ground cinnamon
- 1 cup fresh raspberries

Instructions:

Prepare the cauliflower grits.

In a medium saucepan, heat the cauliflower grits, coconut milk, and maple syrup over medium heat until hot.

Reduce the heat to low and stir in the coconut flour, collagen peptides (if using), vanilla, and cinnamon.

Divide the mixture among bowls or meal prep containers and top with raspberries.

7. Chia Seed Pudding

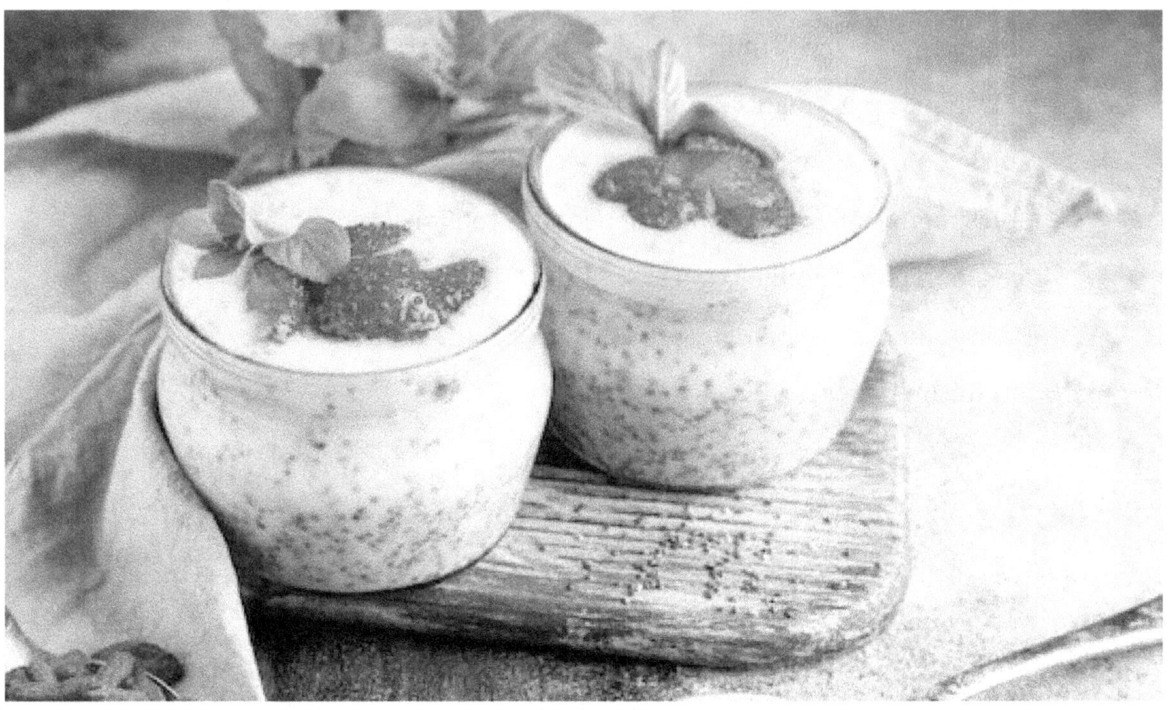

Chia Seed Pudding is a nutritious delight, bursting with health benefits. This delectable treat blends chia seeds, almond milk, and a touch of honey. Packed with omega-3 fatty acids, fiber, and antioxidants, it promotes heart health and aids digestion.

Cooking time: 15 minutes

Servings: 2

Ingredients:

- ¼ cup chia seeds
- 1 cup coconut milk
- ¼ tsp vanilla essence
- 1 tsp honey
- 1 handful of berries

Instructions:

In a bowl, combine chia seeds with warm milk and honey.

Add the rest of the ingredients and pour into a pot.

Cook on low heat for 12-15 minutes.

When ready, remove from heat and serve.

8. Paleo Pancakes

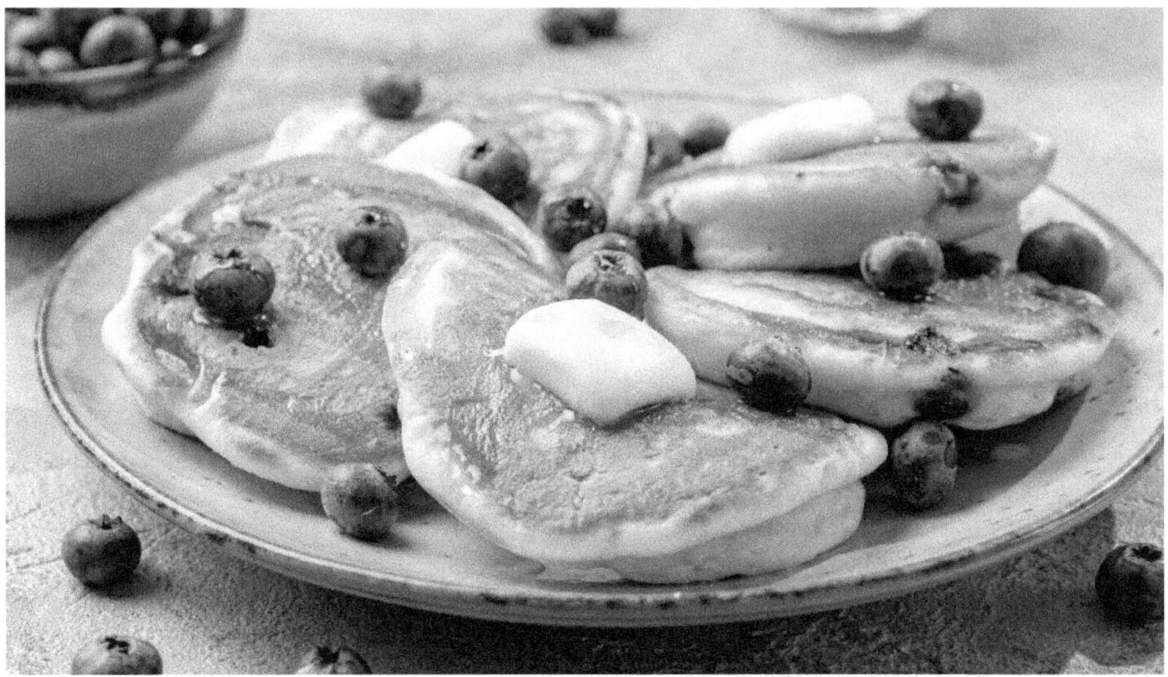

Jumping out of bed is easy when pancakes are part of the morning plan. These pancakes can be made vegan-appropriate by using Non-Dairy Flax Eggs, though the batter may require more liquid. This will give the pancakes a crunchier texture and add omega-3 fatty acids to the nutritional profile.

Cooking time: 40 minutes

Servings: 6

Ingredients:

- ¼ teaspoon salt
- 1 cup tapioca flour
- ½ cup coconut milk
- 1 cup coconut flour
- ½ teaspoon baking powder
- ½ teaspoon baking soda
- 3 large eggs
- 1 teaspoon vanilla extract
- 1½ tablespoons coconut oil, divided

Instructions:

In a mixing bowl, combine the tapioca flour, baking powder, coconut flour, baking soda, and salt.

In another bowl, whisk together the eggs, coconut milk, and vanilla.

Add the wet ingredients to the flour mixture and stir to form a batter.

Heat a large nonstick skillet or griddle over medium heat.

Pour in ½ tablespoon of coconut oil. Tilt the skillet to spread the oil.

Using a spoon or small ladle, drop ¼ cup of batter per pancake into the skillet to make 2 pancakes at a time. Cook for 2 to 3 minutes, or until bubbles form and the bottom has browned.

Flip the pancakes, and cook for 2 to 3 minutes, or until cooked through.

Use the remaining 1 tablespoon of coconut oil in the skillet as needed to cook the rest of the batter. Remove from the heat.

Chapter 2: Fish and Seafood Recipes

9. Baked Ginger-Turmeric–Rubbed Salmon

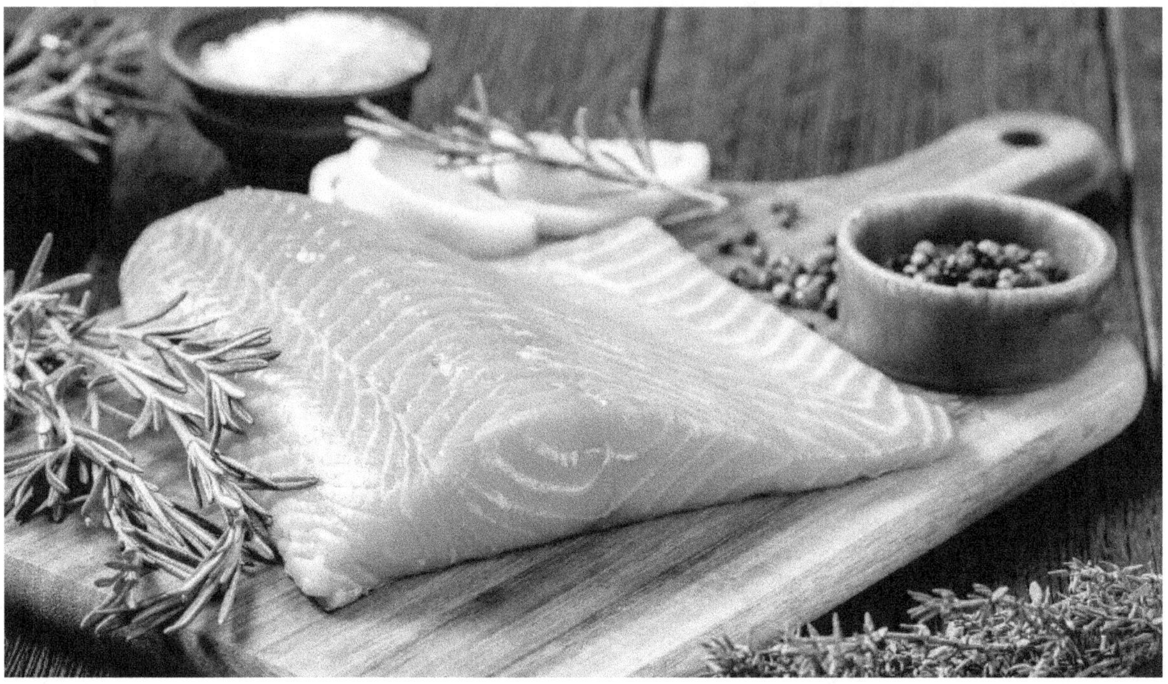

Eating fish twice a week is suggested to lower the risk of heart disease and to help prevent dementia. Try not to eat it battered or fried. Ginger-Turmeric Rub is used in this recipe, which is a thyroid-friendly seasoning that can be used in all three thyroid protocol diets.

Cooking time: 20 minutes

Servings: 4

Ingredients:

- 1½ tablespoons Ginger-Turmeric Rub
- 4 (4-ounce) salmon fillets
- 1 tablespoon coconut oil, melted

Instructions:

Preheat the oven to 400°F. Line a 9-by-13-inch baking pan with parchment paper or aluminum foil.

Rub the ginger-turmeric rub on the salmon.

Place the salmon on the prepared baking pan. Drizzle with the oil.

Transfer the baking pan to the oven and bake for 20 minutes, or until the salmon flakes easily. Remove from the oven. Serve with a favorite salad or side dish.

10. Marinated Grilled Shrimp

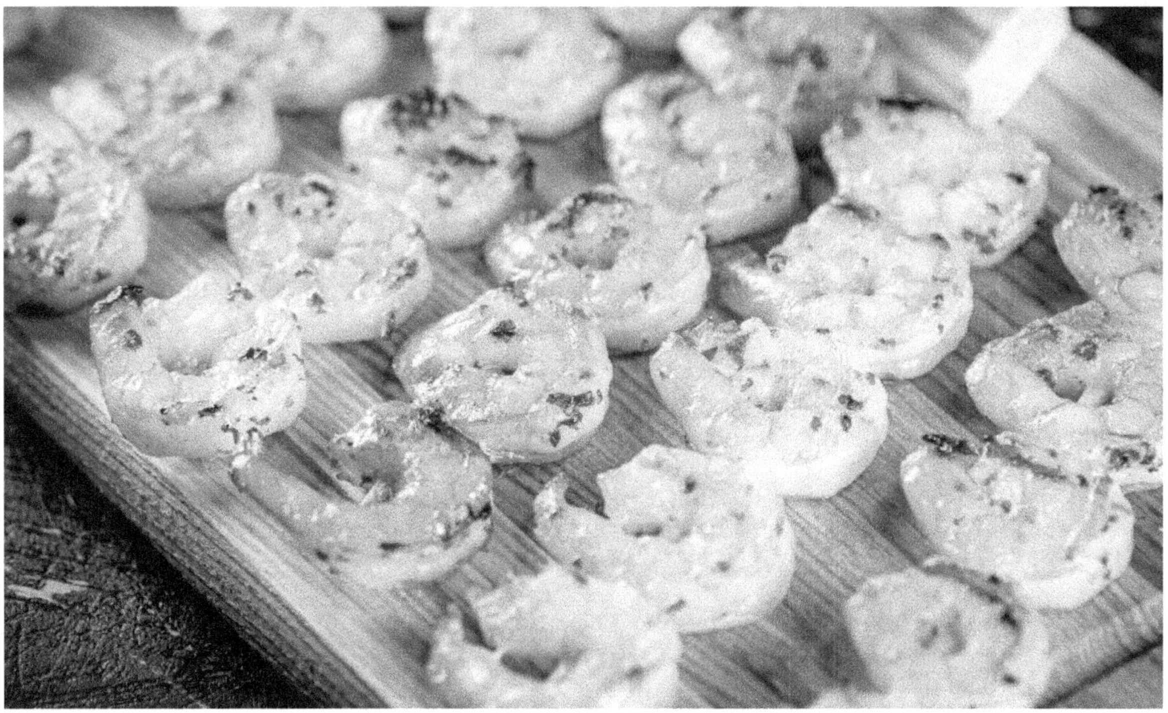

These plump, tender shrimp are marinated in a zesty blend of garlic, and herbs before hitting the grill. Loaded with lean protein, shrimp is a low-calorie, heart-healthy option.

Cooking time: 6 minutes

Servings: 6

Ingredients:

- 3 cloves of garlic, minced
- 1/3 cup extra virgin olive oil
- ¼ cup tomato sauce
- 2 tbsp red wine vinegar
- 2 tbsp fresh basil, chopped
- ½ tsp salt
- ¼ tsp cayenne pepper
- 2 pounds fresh shrimp, deveined and peeled
- ½ cup Skewers

Instructions:

Preheat the grill

Mix all the ingredients together in a large bowl. Make sure the shrimp is well coated. Cover and keep in the refrigerator for about 30 minutes to 1 hour. Stir only once.

Arrange shrimp on skewers by piercing through from the tail to the head. Discard leftover marinade

Lightly oil the grates of the grill and arrange shrimps on it. Grill both sides until shrimp turn opaque. This may take about 5-6 minutes.

Serve and enjoy.

11. Pan-Seared Salmon over Arugula with Yellow Beets

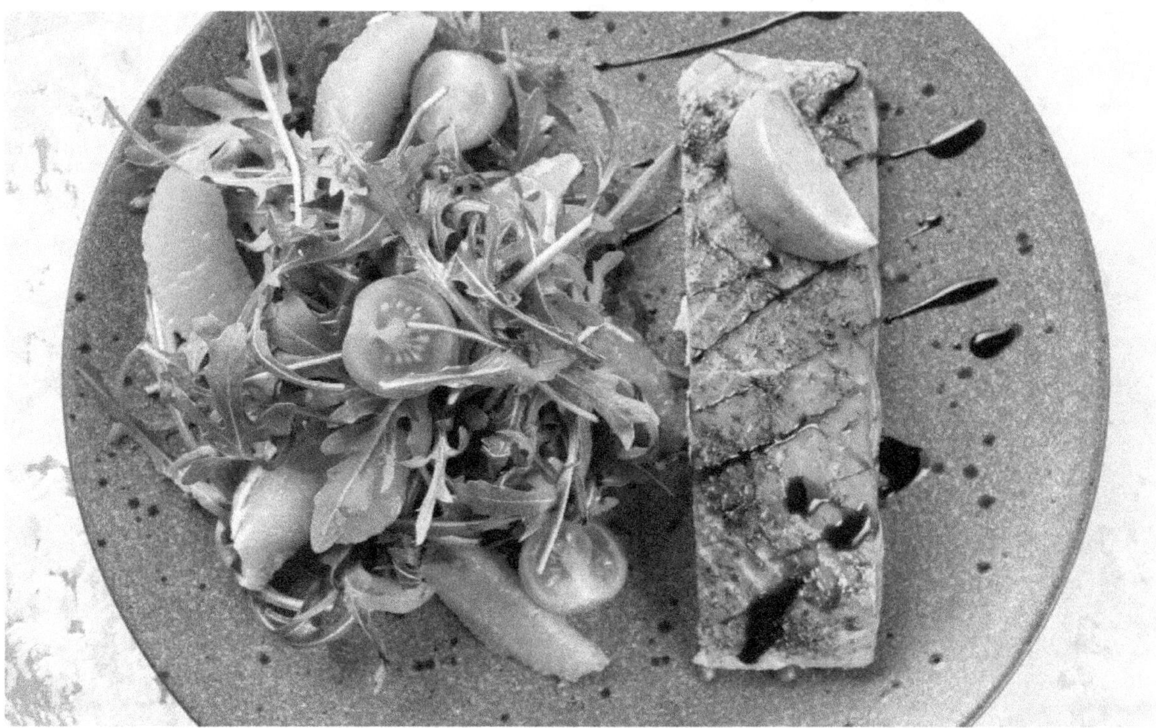

Searing meat or fish is a method of cooking that results in a crispy texture on the outside and tender quality on the inside. This is a great dish to serve any time of year but is particularly tasty in the summer when craving a delicious salad. Salmon provides protein and anti-inflammatory omega-3 fatty acids.

Cooking time: 60 minutes

Servings: 4

Ingredients:

- 4 medium yellow beets, scrubbed
- 2 tablespoons extra-virgin olive oil, divided
- 1 teaspoon salt, plus more as needed
- 4 (4-ounce) salmon fillets
- 1 teaspoon freshly ground black pepper
- 1 (10-ounce) bag arugula
- 1 cup Apple Cider Vinaigrette

Instructions:

Preheat the oven to 400°F. Line a 15-by-12-inch baking pan with aluminum foil.

Cut the tops and ends off the beets. Place in the prepared baking pan. Drizzle 1 tablespoon of oil over the beets and dust with the salt.

Transfer the baking pan to the oven and roast for 45 minutes. Remove from the oven. Let the beets cool for 10 minutes.

Once the beets have cooled, peel the skins off, and slice the beets into thin rounds.

While the beets roast, in a large nonstick skillet, heat the remaining 1 tablespoon of oil over high heat.

Season the salmon with salt and the pepper. Add to the skillet and cook for 5 to 7 minutes per side, or until it flakes easily and has completely cooked. Remove from the heat.

Put the arugula and sliced beets in a large salad bowl. Dress with the vinaigrette. Toss the salad. Divide among 4 bowls.

Top each serving with the salmon.

12. Chili-Lime Shrimp Fajitas

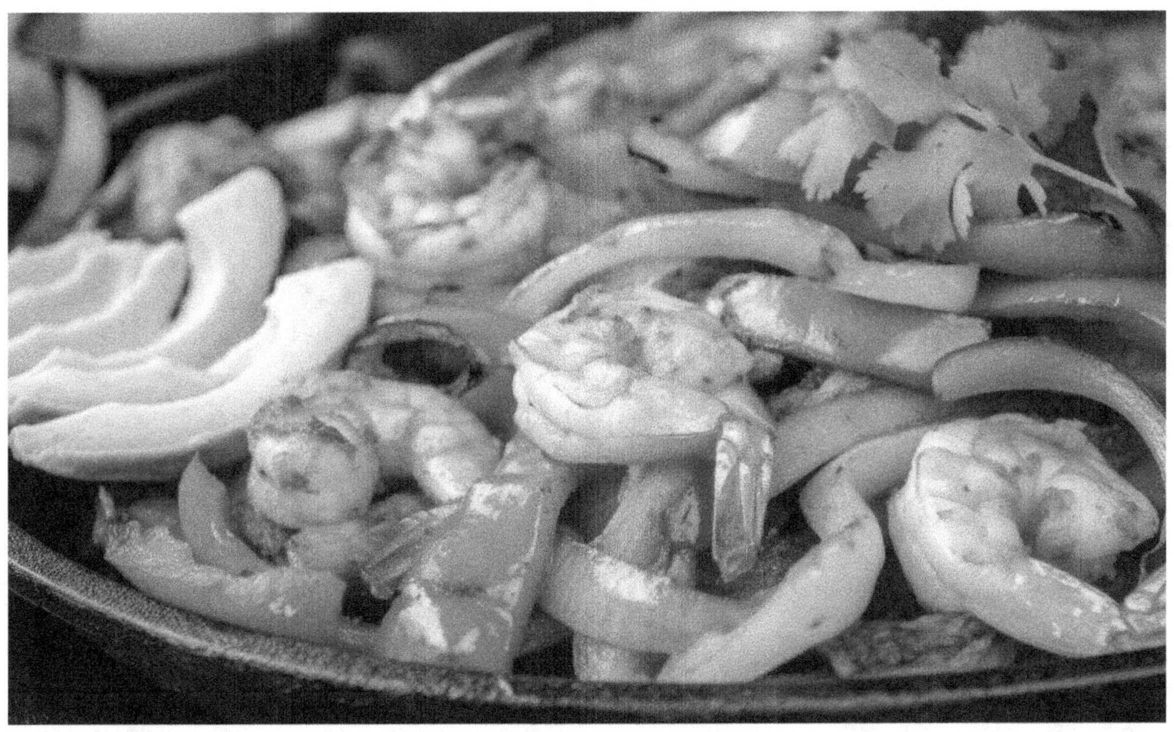

These shrimp fajitas will bring a bold taste to your next meal. Served in a chili-lime vinaigrette, this dish has the Mexican flavor you love without any ingredients you don't have. Shrimp, a high-protein shellfish, contains many important nutrients including selenium.

Cooking time: 6 minutes

Servings: 4

Ingredients:

- 1 tablespoon extra-virgin olive oil
- 1-pound raw shrimp, peeled and deveined
- ¼ teaspoon salt
- ¼ teaspoon freshly ground black pepper
- ½ cup Chili-Lime Vinaigrette
- 8 grain-free tortillas, or lettuce leaves
- 1 cup shredded lettuce of choice
- ½ cup diced avocado
- 2 tablespoons diced red onion
- 1 tablespoon finely minced fresh cilantro

Instructions:

In a medium skillet over medium heat, heat the olive oil.

Next, add the shrimp, salt, and pepper. Cook for 2 to 3 minutes, stirring occasionally, or until the shrimp are pink and no longer translucent. Remove the shrimp from the pan and set aside.

Add the vinaigrette to the skillet. Cook for 2 to 3 minutes.

Return the shrimp to the pan and gently toss to mix in the sauce. Serve inside the tortillas or lettuce leaves, topped with lettuce, avocado, red onion, and cilantro.

13. Seared Sea Scallops with Avocado Cream

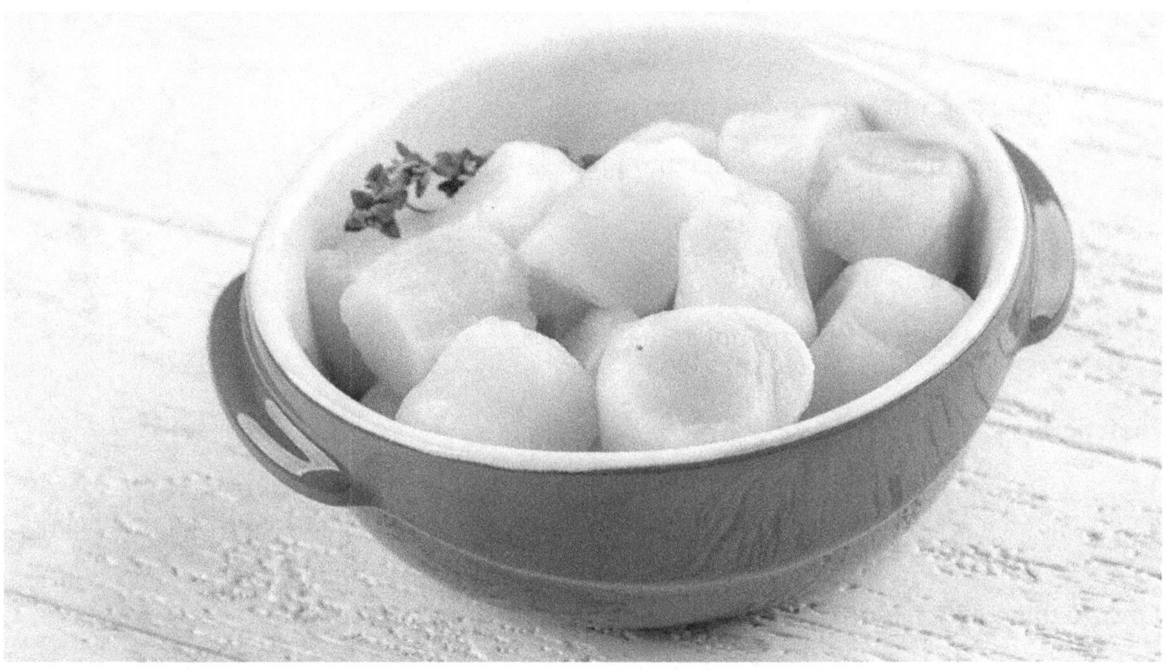

This delightful dish, Seared Sea Scallops with Avocado Cream, offers a perfect blend of flavors and nutrients. Tender, succulent sea scallops are expertly seared to a golden perfection, creating a crispy exterior that contrasts beautifully with the creamy, velvety avocado cream.

Cooking time: 20 minutes

Servings: 4

Ingredients:

- 1-pound fresh sea scallops
- ¼ teaspoon salt
- ¼ teaspoon freshly ground black pepper
- 1 teaspoon freshly squeezed lemon juice
- ¼ teaspoon fresh thyme leaves
- 2 tablespoons coconut oil
- ½ cup Avocado Cream Sauce

Instructions:

Gently pat the scallops dry with a paper towel and season both sides with salt and pepper.

Drizzle them with lemon juice and sprinkle with the thyme.

In a cast-iron skillet over medium-high heat, heat the coconut oil for 2 minutes.

Once hot, gently place the scallops in the skillet. Cook the scallops for 2 minutes. Flip and cook for 90 seconds more.

Top with the avocado cream sauce and serve immediately.

14. Crispy Baked Cod Fingers

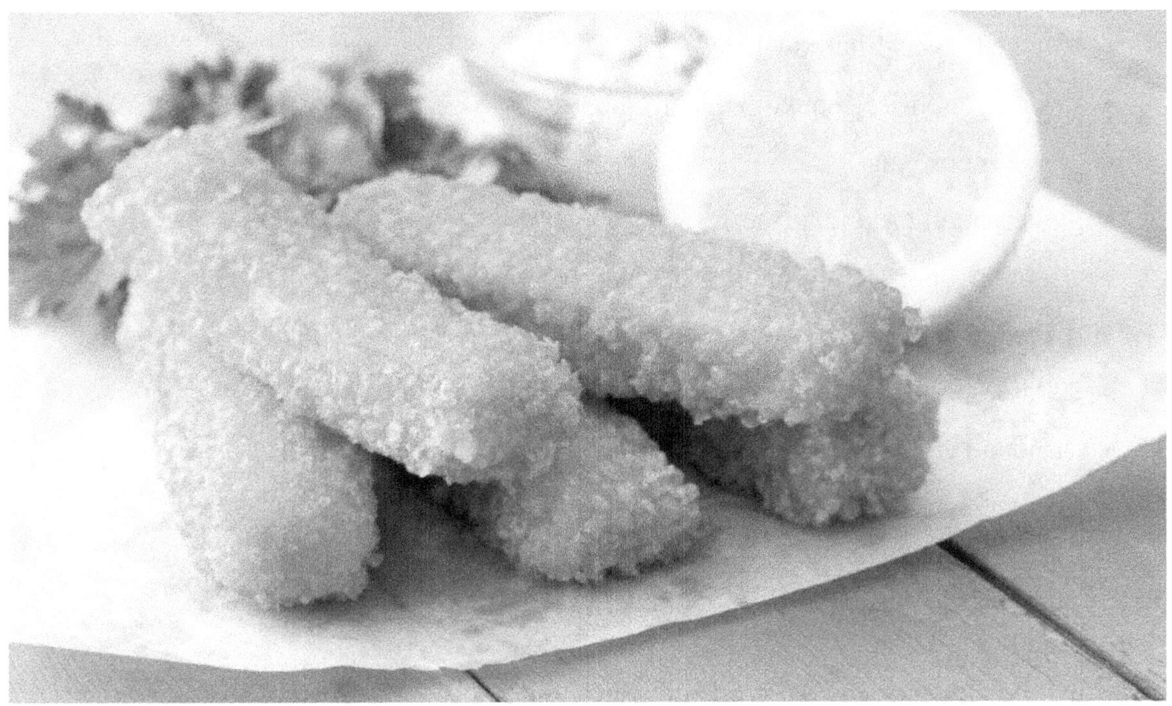

This recipe is a wholesome treat that's sure to please both your taste buds and your health-conscious conscience.

Cooking time: 20 minutes

Servings: 4

Ingredients:

- ¼ cup ground flaxseed
- 3 tablespoons filtered water
- 1 cup gluten-free panko bread crumbs
- ½ teaspoon salt
- ½ teaspoon ground turmeric
- ¼ teaspoon freshly ground black pepper
- ¼ teaspoon garlic powder
- 2 tablespoons extra-virgin olive oil
- 1 pound cod fillets, cut into 1-by-1-by-4-inch strips, patted dry
- ½ cup Avocado Cream Sauce

Instructions:

In a small bowl, whisk the flaxseed and water. Set aside.

In a medium bowl, stir together the bread crumbs, salt, turmeric, pepper, and garlic powder.

In a cast-iron skillet over medium-high heat, heat the olive oil for 1 to 2 minutes until hot.

Dredge the cod fingers in the flaxseed and water mixture, then dredge in the bread crumb mixture. Carefully place in the hot oil. Cook for 2 to 3 minutes until golden brown. Flip and cook for 2 to 3 minutes more until golden brown. Carefully transfer to paper towels to drain.

Serve immediately with the avocado cream sauce for dipping.

15. King Prawn & Garlicky Spinach

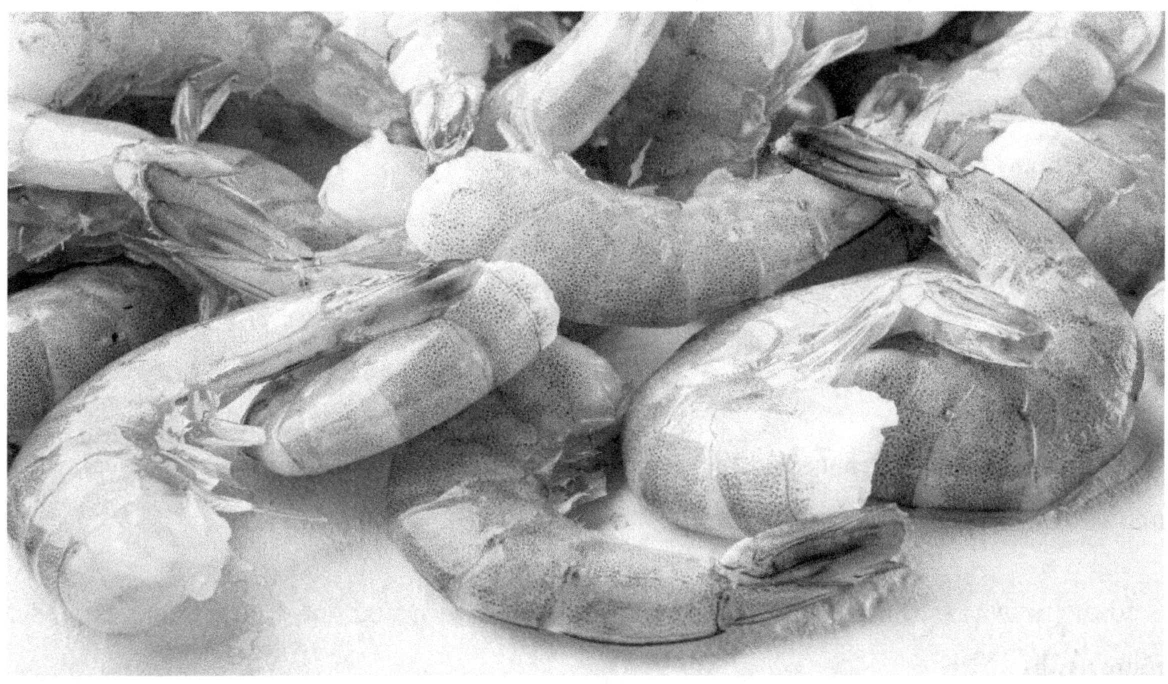

This delectable combo provides a wealth of essential nutrients. King prawns offer a protein punch, while spinach delivers vitamins A and C, iron, and fiber.

Cooking time: 30 minutes

Servings: 4

Ingredients:

- 1 lb. king prawns (shrimps), shelled
- 7 oz spinach leaves, washed
- 4 tomatoes, chopped
- 4 spring onions (scallions), chopped
- 3 cloves of garlic, crushed
- 2 tablespoons olive oil

Instructions:

Heat the oil in a frying pan, add the tomatoes, 1 clove of garlic, spring onions (scallions) and cook for 4-5 minutes.

Add the prawns (shrimps) and cook until they are pink throughout. Remove them and set them aside.

Add the spinach and the remaining garlic to the pan and cook until the spinach has wilted. You can add a little hot water or oil to the pan if you need extra moisture.

Serve the spinach onto plates and add the prawn mixture on top. Serve and eat straight away.

16. Marinated Tuna Steak

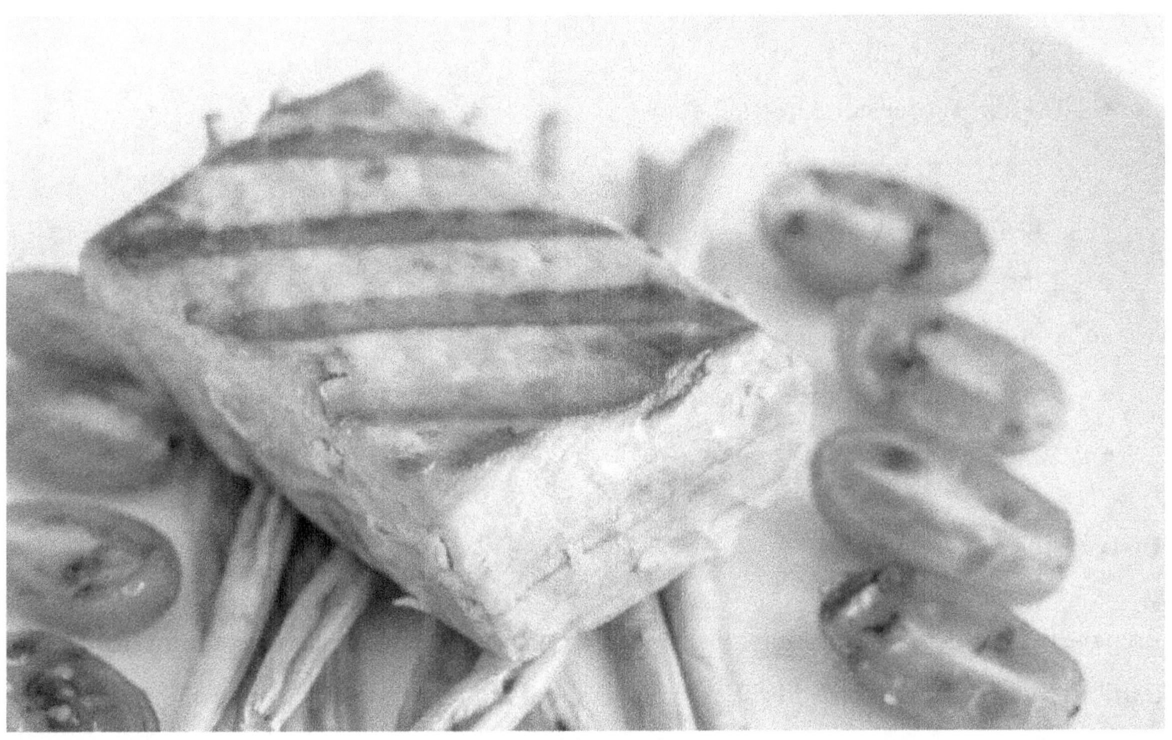

This protein-packed dish boasts a burst of flavors, marrying the ocean's bounty with zesty marinade. Tuna, rich in omega-3 fatty acids, supports heart health and brain function.

Cooking time: 50 minutes

Servings: 4

Ingredients:

- 4 tuna steaks (4 oz each)
- 1/4 cup of orange juice
- 1/4 cup Worcestershire sauce
- 2 tbsp extra virgin olive oil
- 1 tbsp lemon juice
- 2 tbsp fresh parsley, chopped
- 1 clove garlic, minced
- 1/2 tsp chopped fresh oregano
- 1/2 tsp ground black pepper

Instructions:

Prepare the marinade by mixing all the ingredients except the tuna in a medium bowl. Mix until well combined, then add the tuna steaks and coat all sides. Leave in the refrigerator for 30 minutes to marinade.

While waiting, preheat the grill and lightly oil the grates.

Remove tuna and marinade from the refrigerator. Arrange tuna steaks on the grates and grill. Cook for 5 minutes, then turn tuna steaks and coat with marinade. Turn the tuna periodically and baste with marinade until steak is grilled to the desired level. Discard leftover marinade

Serve and enjoy.

Chapter 3: Poultry Recipes

17. Sundried Tomato Chicken & Mushrooms

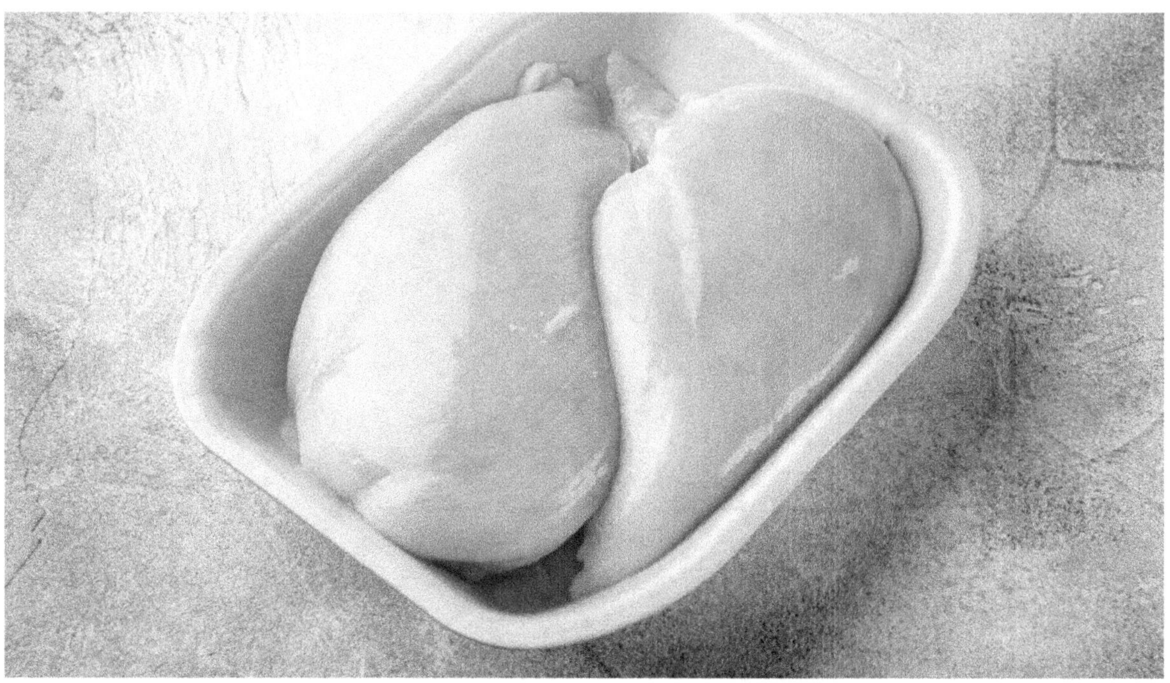

Packed with protein, it fuels your muscles, while the tomatoes offer a dose of antioxidants and vitamins. Mushrooms add a rich umami flavor, along with essential minerals.

Cooking time: 25 minutes

Servings: 4

Ingredients:

- 7oz mushrooms, sliced
- 4 chicken breasts
- 8 large sundried tomatoes, finely chopped
- 2 tablespoons chives, chopped
- 2 tablespoons olive oil
- 2 garlic cloves, chopped finely
- 1 bag of mixed salad leaves

Instructions:

Place the tomatoes into a bowl and add the chives and garlic. Mix well.

Make a horizontal incision in each of the chicken breasts and press some of the tomato mixture into them.

Heat the oil in a frying pan and add the chicken. Cook for around 6 minutes on each side. Add in the mushrooms towards the end of cooking and cook until they have softened.

Scatter some mixed salad leaves onto plates and serve the chicken and mushrooms. Eat straight away.

18. Easy Chicken Lasagna

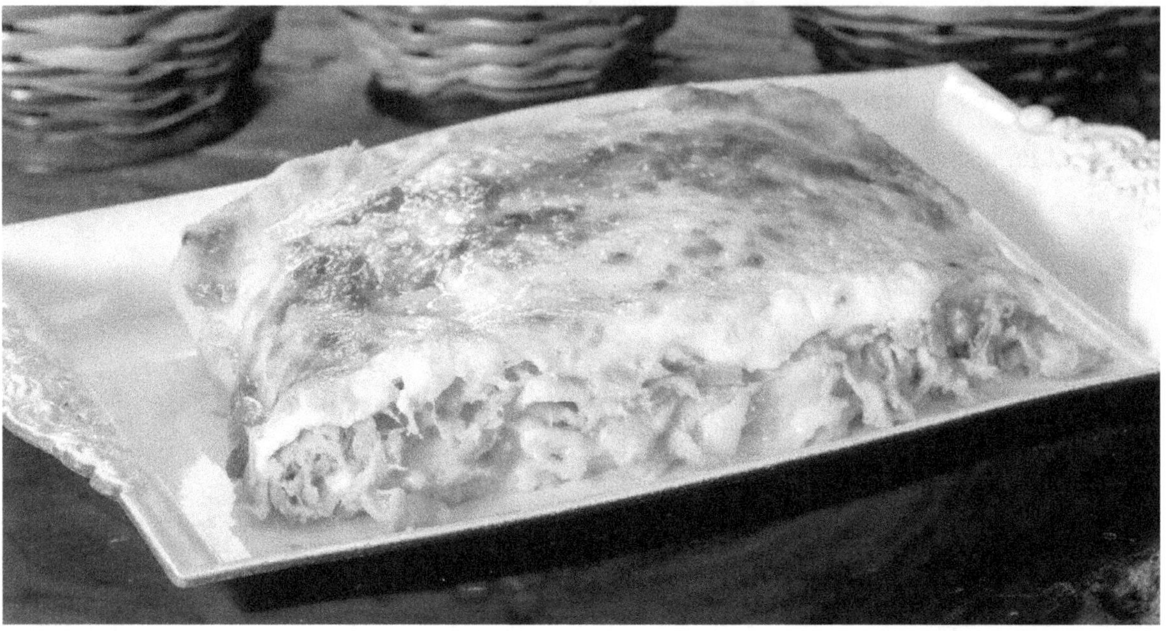

This delectable Easy Chicken Lasagna is a wholesome meal bursting with flavor. Perfect for busy weeknights, this dish is a tasty way to nourish your body and delight your taste buds.

Cooking time: 1 hour 20 minutes

Servings: 9

Ingredients:

- 1-pound chicken breast, shredded
- 1/2 pound white mushrooms, thinly sliced
- 26 oz fat-free marinara sauce
- 2 large egg whites, lightly whisked
- 16 oz part-skim mozzarella cheese, shredded
- 1/4 cup Parmigiano-Reggiano cheese, grated
- 1/2 tsp fresh nutmeg, grated
- 8 oz no-salt-added tomato sauce
- 15 oz fat-free ricotta cheese
- 9 oz no-boil lasagna noodles
- Non-stick spray

Instructions:

Preheat the oven to 375°F.

Spray the non-stick spray on a large saucepan and place over medium heat. Add the chicken and cook until all sides are lightly browned. This may take 3-4 minutes.

Add in the mushrooms. Cook until the liquid comes out or for 5 minutes.

Pour in the marina sauce, stir, lower the heat and allow to simmer. Set the pot aside

Mix the mozzarella and ricotta cheese, nutmeg, and egg whites in a small bowl. Set aside.

Spread the tomato sauce mixture smoothly on the bottom of a baking pan. Arrange 5 lasagna noodles over the sauce in the first layer. Add 1/3 of the chicken mixture.

Repeat step 6 until the ingredients are exhausted. (The ingredients listed above will only make 3 layers).

Sprinkle Parmigiano-Reggiano on top of the lasagna, cover, then bake for 45 minutes.

Uncover, then bake until the top turns slightly brown. This may take about 10 minutes.

Allow cooling for 5 minutes before serving.

19. Turkey & Sweet Potato Pie

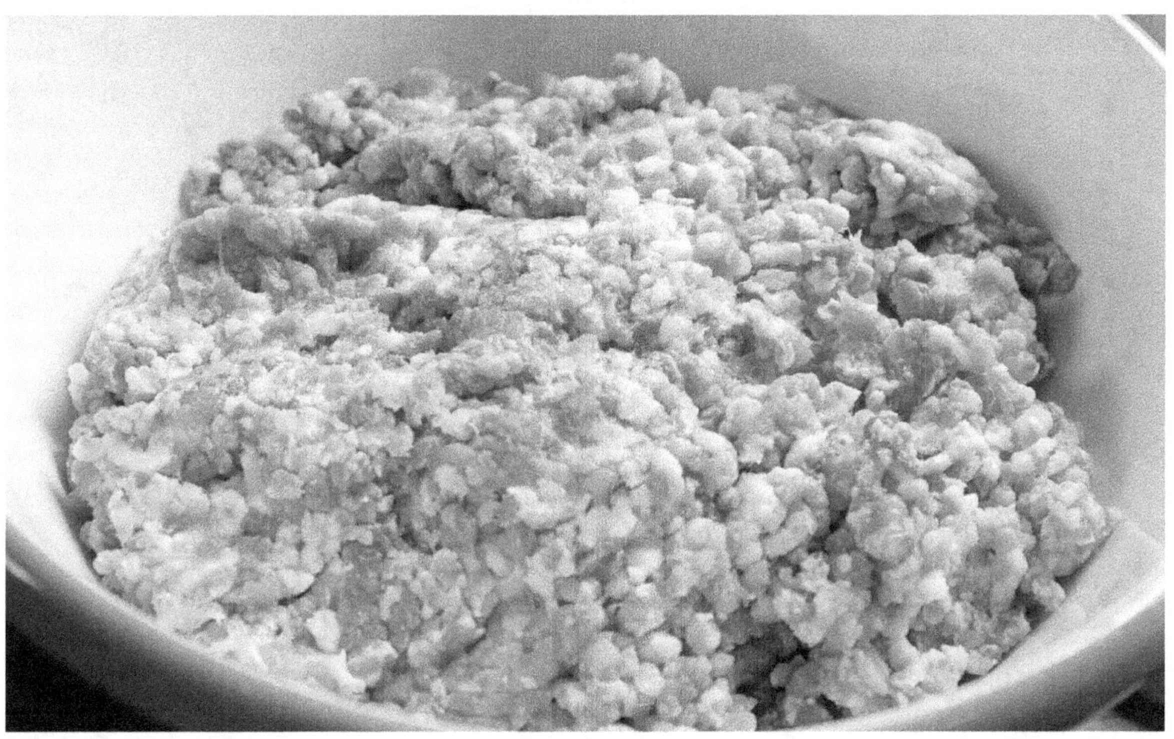

This Turkey & Sweet Potato Pie is a nutritious delight, packing a punch of protein and essential vitamins. Succulent turkey pairs perfectly with creamy sweet potatoes, creating a mouthwatering marriage of flavors.

Cooking time: 50 minutes

Servings: 4

Ingredients:

- 1 lb. (5 oz) sweet potato, peeled and chopped
- 1 lb. minced (ground) turkey
- 14 oz can of chopped tomatoes
- 5 oz frozen peas
- 3 celery stalks, finely chopped
- 1 onion, finely chopped
- 1 large carrot, peeled, finely chopped
- 2 tablespoons tomato purée (paste)
- 1 teaspoon dried mixed herbs
- 1 tablespoon olive oil
- 2 teaspoons Worcestershire sauce
- Sea salt
- Freshly ground black pepper

Instructions:

Heat the oil in a saucepan, add the carrot, onion and celery and cook gently for around 5 minutes until the vegetables have softened.

Add the turkey mince and brown it for around 5 minutes. Stir in the tomato purée (paste), Worcestershire sauce, tomatoes, peas and herbs. Cook for around 20 minutes, stirring occasionally.

In the meantime, boil the sweet potato in water for around 8-10 minutes or until it becomes tender. Drain off the excess water and mash the sweet potato until smooth. Season it with salt and pepper.

Spoon the turkey mixture into an ovenproof dish then add the mashed sweet potato on top, smoothing it out to the sides.

Transfer it to the oven and cook for 30 minutes at 180C/360F.

20. Herbaceous Chicken Meatballs

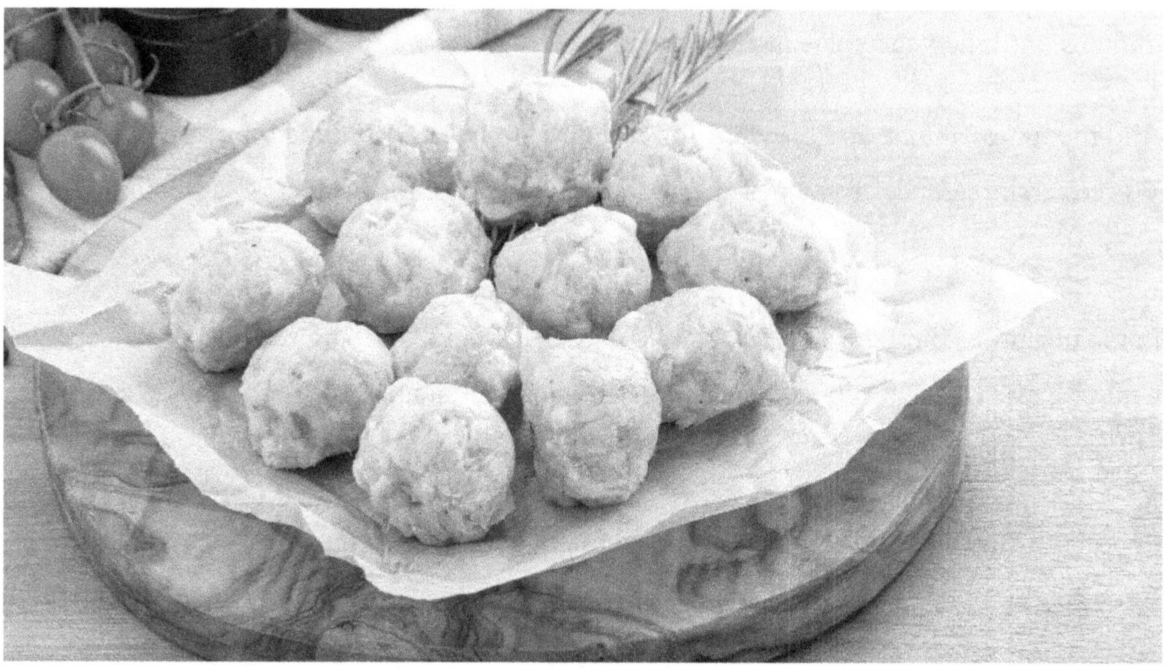

These juicy meatballs are bursting with flavor thanks to the fresh herbs. They will fill your entire kitchen with the warm aromas of ginger, garlic, soy sauce–like coconut aminos, and spicy black pepper. You can easily customize these with different herbs to mimic the tastes of your favorite cuisine.

Cooking time: 30 minutes

Servings: 4

Ingredients:

- ¼ cup loosely packed finely chopped fresh cilantro
- 3 tablespoons finely minced yellow onion
- 2 tablespoons finely minced celery
- 2 tablespoons coconut aminos
- 1 tablespoon freshly squeezed lime juice
- 1 tablespoon finely minced garlic
- ½ tablespoon minced peeled fresh ginger
- ¼ teaspoon salt
- ¼ teaspoon freshly ground black pepper
- 3 tablespoons cassava flour
- 1 pound ground chicken
- 1 tablespoon extra-virgin olive oil

Instructions:

Preheat the oven to 400°F.

In a large bowl, combine the cilantro, onion, celery, coconut aminos, lime juice, garlic, ginger, salt, and pepper. Mix well.

Stir in the cassava flour and mix until the ingredients are well incorporated.

Mix in the ground chicken. Using your hands, ensure all the ingredients are well mixed, but be careful not to overmix.

Once mixed, roll into 1½-inch meatballs.

In a large oven-safe skillet, heat the olive oil over medium-high heat. Carefully place the meatballs in the pan and cook for 3 to 5 minutes, until browned on one side. Flip the meatballs and cook for another 3 to 5 minutes, until browned.

Place the pan in the oven and cook for an additional 10 minutes, or until an internal temperature of 165°F is reached and the juices run clear.

21. Chicken, Cilantro, and Cucumber Wraps

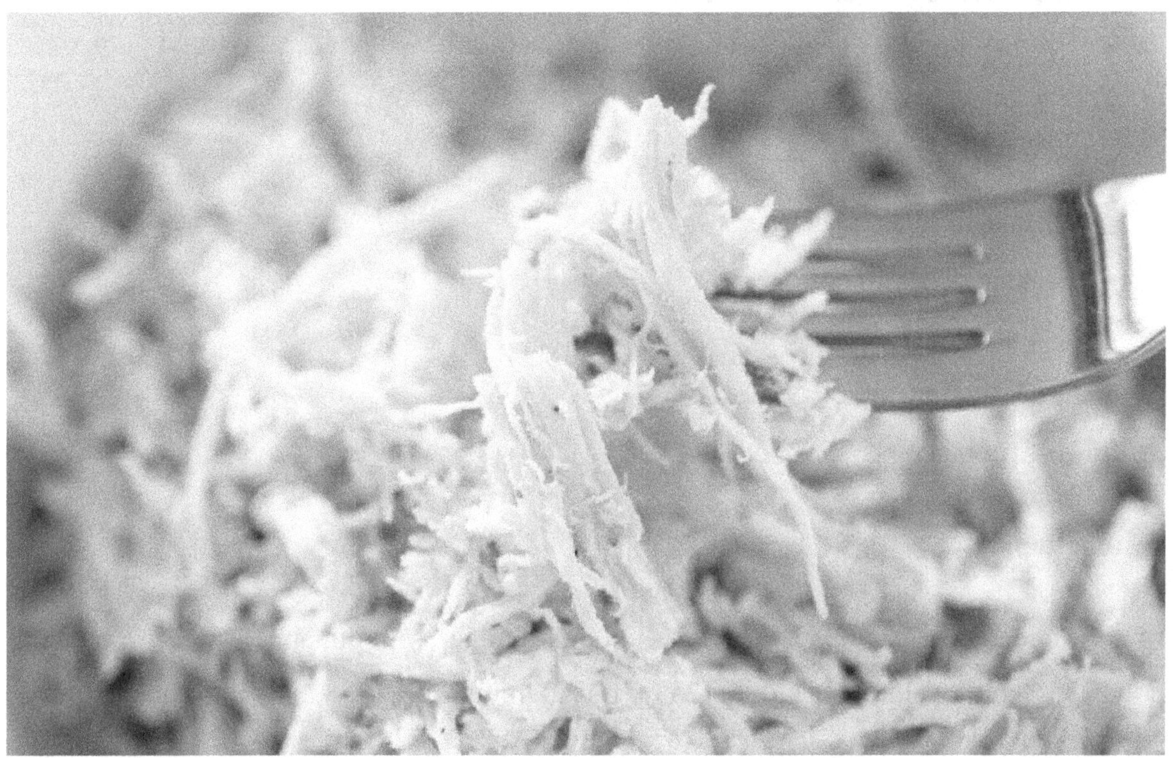

These wraps are a nutrient powerhouse, supplying vitamins A, C, and K, along with minerals like potassium and magnesium. Low in calories and high in fiber, they're an excellent choice for those looking to maintain a nutritious diet.

Cooking time: 35 minutes

Servings: 4

Ingredients:

- 2 cups shredded cooked chicken breast
- 1/4 cup low-fat mayonnaise
- 1 tsp ginger, minced
- 1/4 cup cilantro, chopped
- 4 flour tortillas, 8 inches
- 1 tsp dark sesame oil
- 1/4 tsp salt
- 1 medium cucumber, diced
- 1/4 tsp black pepper

Instructions:

Mix the cucumber, mayonnaise, chicken, cilantro, ginger, salt, oil, and pepper in a medium bowl. Toss until well combined. Set aside for 10 minutes to allow flavors to blend.

Place a large non-stick skillet over medium heat and toast the tortillas. Make sure both sides are accounted for. Remove from heat after 2 minutes.

Share the chicken filling equally among the tortillas and roll them up. Divide the rolls into equal halves.

Serve and enjoy.

22. Curry Chicken with Spinach

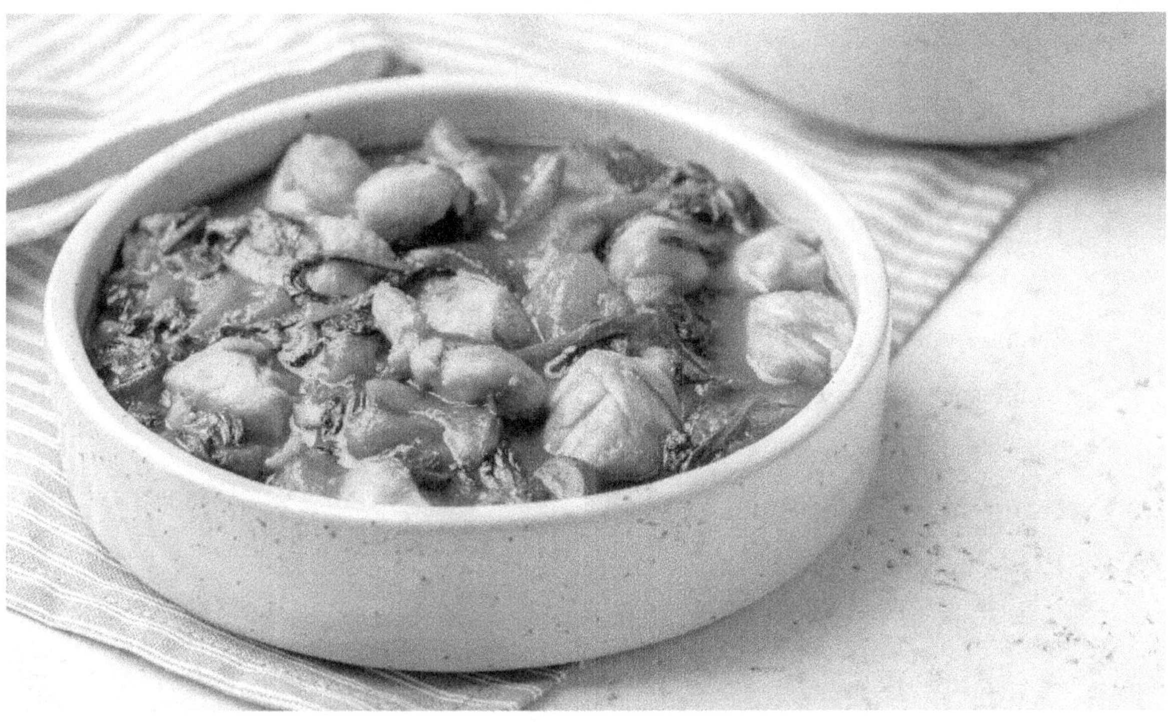

There's something comforting about chicken curry. Is it the warm spice? The savory sauce? Whatever it is, this delicious Paleo-friendly dish is irresistible.

Cooking time: 30 minutes

Servings: 4

Ingredients:

- 1 pound skinless boneless chicken thighs
- ½ teaspoon salt
- ½ teaspoon freshly ground black pepper
- 1 tablespoon olive oil
- 1 small onion, chopped
- 1 red bell pepper, cored and thinly sliced
- 2 cups spinach, ripped
- 2 tablespoons curry powder
- 2 garlic cloves, minced
- 1 cup Chicken Bone Broth
- 1 (15-ounce) can tomato sauce

Instructions:

Season the chicken thighs with salt and pepper.

In a large skillet, heat the oil over medium heat.

Add the chicken and cook for 6 to 8 minutes, or until lightly browned, then place on a large plate.

To the same skillet, add the onion, bell pepper, and spinach. Cook for 3 to 4 minutes, or until the onion is soft.

Add the curry powder and garlic. Toss the vegetables to coat.

Increase the heat to high. Add the broth, tomato sauce, and chicken. Boil for 1 minute.

Reduce the heat to a simmer. Cover and cook for 4 to 5 minutes, until the chicken has fully cooked. Remove from the heat and serve.

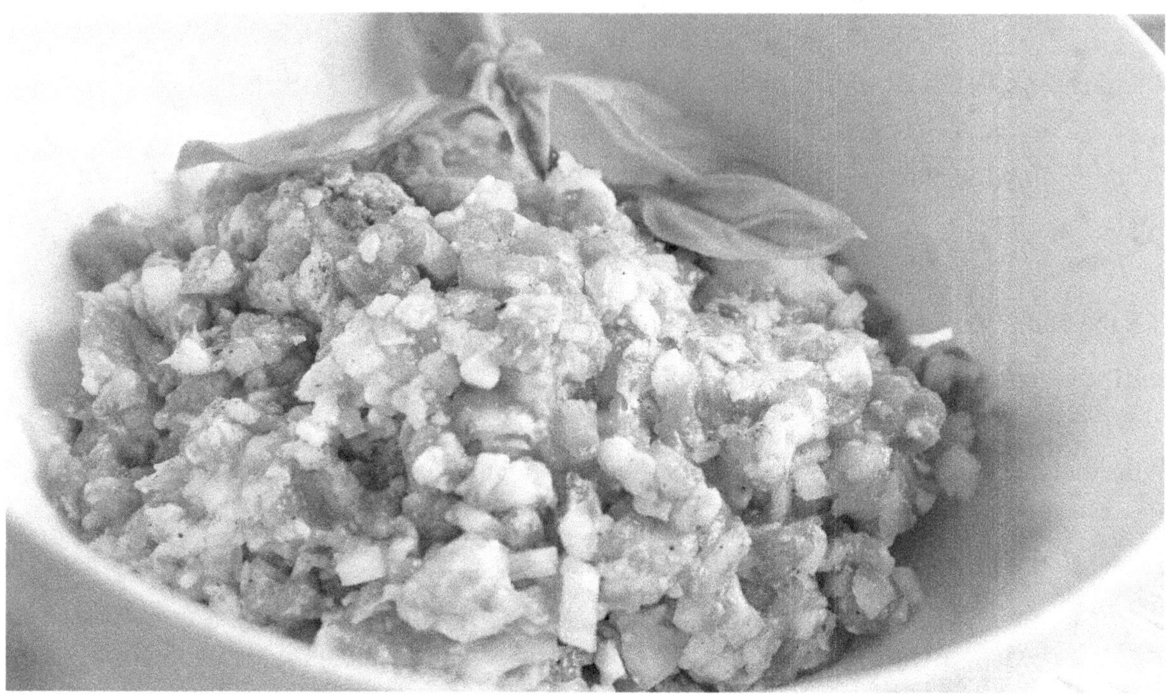

These Thai Turkey Burger Wraps are a nutrient-packed delight. Ground turkey, rich in lean protein, forms the base. A harmonious blend of taste and health, these wraps are a delightful addition to your dinner repertoire.

Cooking time: 25 minutes

Servings: 4

Ingredients:

- 1 lb. minced (ground) turkey
- 3 garlic cloves, crushed
- 2 large tomatoes, diced
- 2 inner stalks lemongrass, finely chopped
- 2 carrots, peeled and grated
- 1 onion, finely chopped
- 1 large bunch coriander (cilantro), finely chopped
- 1 tablespoon fish sauce
- 1 tablespoon chopped fresh coriander (cilantro)
- Few heads baby gem lettuce

Instructions:

Place the turkey mince, garlic, coriander (cilantro), lemongrass, onion and fish sauce into a bowl and combine them well. Shape the mixture into balls then flatten them into round shapes. Place them on a lightly greased baking tray.

Transfer them to the oven and bake at 200C/400F for 15–20 minutes.

Meanwhile, you can make little salad boats to serve them in.

In a bowl combine the chopped tomatoes with the grated carrots and a few sprigs of coriander (cilantro).

Serve the turkey burgers into the lettuce leaves and add a spoonful of the tomato and carrot mixture into each one. Eat straight away. You could even add a little guacamole or mayonnaise to each one.

Chapter 4: Beef and Pork Recipes

24. Steak & Root Vegetable Casserole

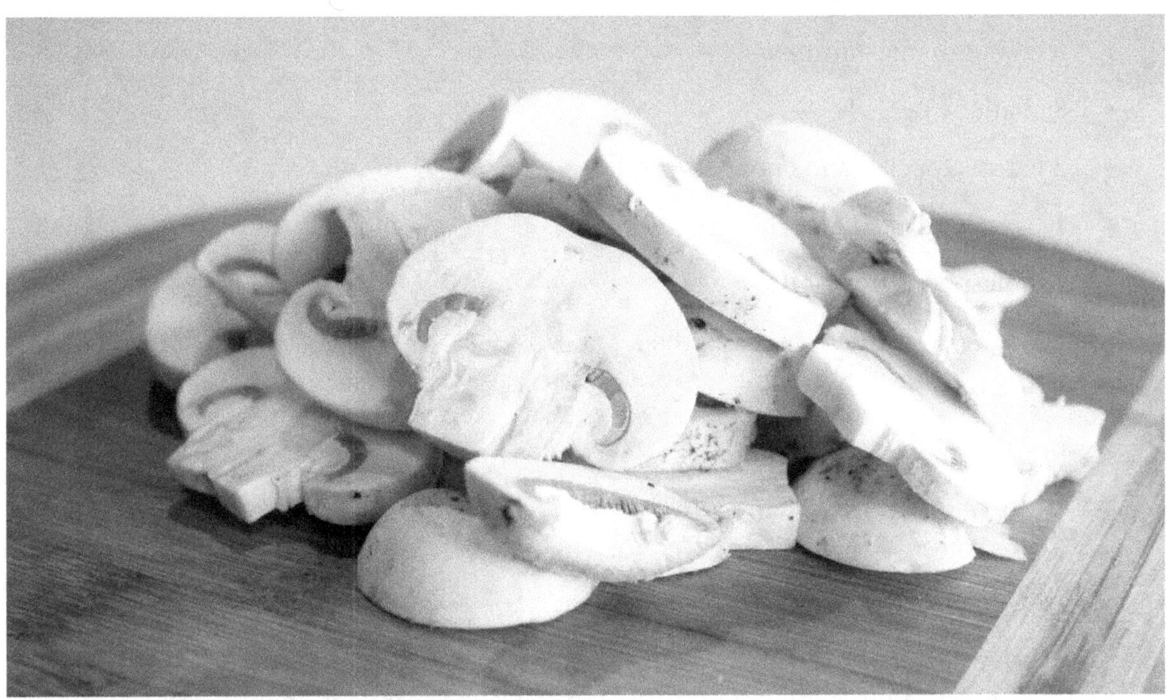

This nutrient-packed dish combines tender chunks of steak with a medley of root vegetables, creating a mouthwatering symphony of flavors. Rich in protein, the steak fuels your muscles, while the carrots, parsnips, and potatoes provide essential vitamins and dietary fiber.

Cooking time: 2 hours

Servings: 4

Ingredients:

- 1½ lb. stewing steak
- 6 oz button mushrooms
- 8 shallots, peeled
- 2 carrots, peeled and chopped
- 1 parsnip, peeled and chopped
- 1 tablespoons olive oil
- 1-2 teaspoons dried mixed herbs
- Sea salt
- Freshly ground black pepper
- 1 pint gluten-free beef stock (broth)

Instructions:

Heat a tablespoon of olive oil in a pan, add the steak and brown it on all sides.

Transfer the steak to an ovenproof dish. Add in the mushrooms, shallots, carrots, parsnip, herbs and stock (broth). Place a lid on the dish or cover it with foil.

Transfer it to the oven and cook at 150C/300F for 1 ½ to 2 hours and the meat should be tender.

Season with salt and pepper. Serve with new potatoes or squash mash.

25. Tender Pork Curry

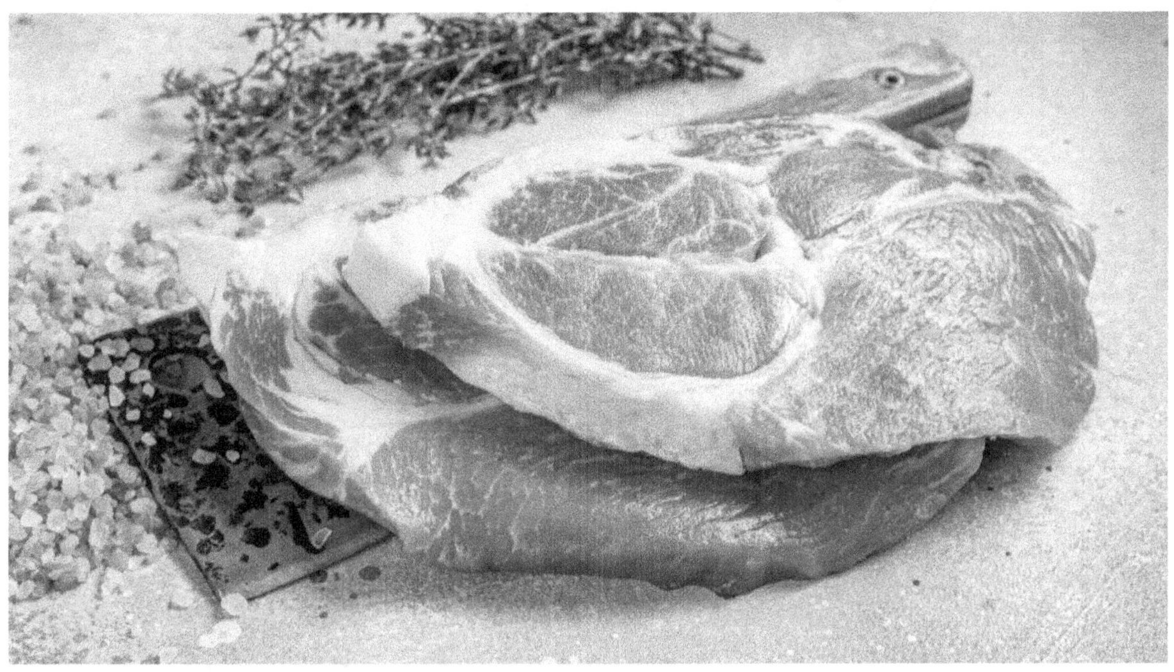

This wholesome dish boasts a rich blend of protein, vitamins, and minerals. Packed with essential nutrients like protein, iron, and vitamins, this curry offers a satisfying and nutritious meal.

Cooking time: 6 hours

Servings: 4

Ingredients:

- 1 lb. pork steaks, cubed
- 14 oz tinned chopped tomatoes
- 5 oz broccoli, broken into florets
- 3 cloves garlic, minced
- 1 onion, chopped
- 1 green chilli, finely chopped
- 1 tablespoon curry powder
- 1 teaspoon ground ginger
- 1 teaspoon ground coriander (cilantro)
- 1 cup gluten-free beef stock (broth)
- 1 tablespoon olive oil
- Sea salt
- Freshly ground black pepper

Instructions:

Heat the olive oil in a frying pan and add in the pork. Brown it for several minutes then transfer it to a slow cooker.

Add in all the remaining ingredients and stir well. Cover the slow cooker and cook for around 6 hours or until the meat is tender. Serve with rice or roast vegetables.

26. Stuffed Banana Peppers

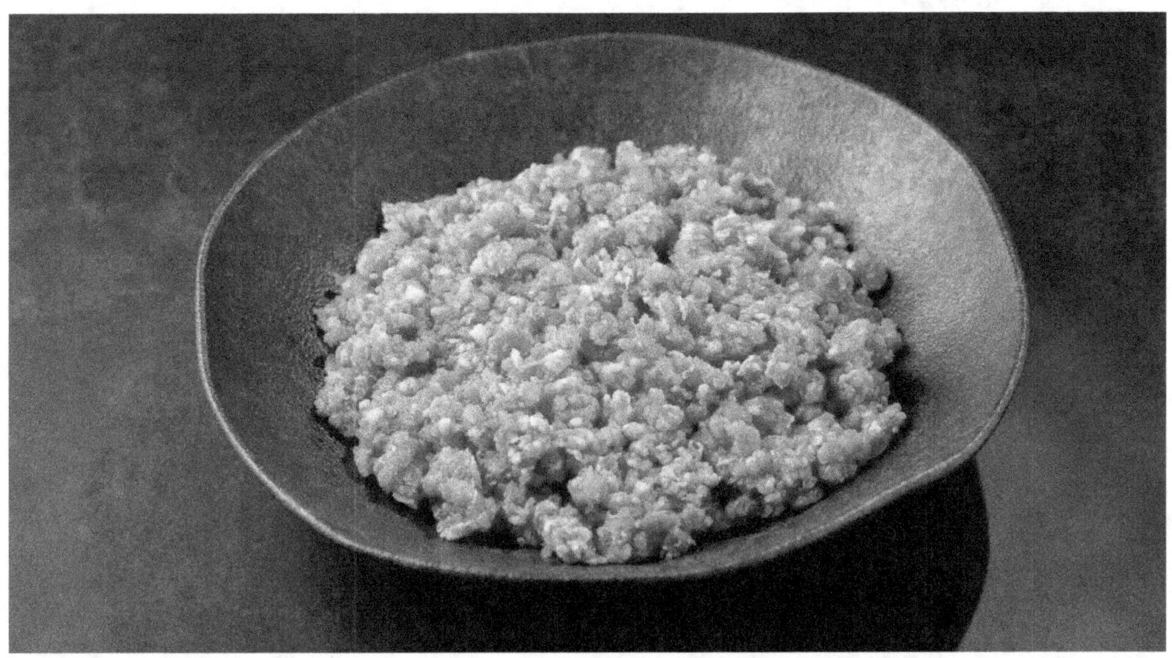

This recipe makes for a satisfying, nutritious meal that's both delicious and beneficial for your body, making it an ideal choice for those seeking a wholesome and flavorsome dinner option.

Cooking time: 40 minutes

Servings: 6

Ingredients:

- 1/4 cup all-purpose flour
- 1-pound extra-lean ground beef (93% lean)
- 12 banana peppers, hot or sweet
- 1 small onion, thinly sliced
- 1 medium egg
- 1/2 cup Swiss cheese, grated
- 1/4 tsp black pepper
- 1/4 tsp vegetable oil.

Instructions:

Preheat the oven to 350°F.

Prepare the peppers by washing and cutting off the top and bottom.

In a medium skillet, brown the beef and onions. This will take about five minutes. When ready, stir in the cheese.

Stuff the beef and cheese mixture into the peppers. Set aside.

Pour flour on a chopping board.

Mix the egg and black pepper in a separate bowl. Dip the peppers into the egg and then roll in flour to coat. Dip into the egg a second time and then coat in flour again.

Coat a baking dish with oil and arrange the peppers in it. Bake for 20 minutes, then remove when the cheese is melted and the flour coating turns brown.

27. Meatballs & Roast Vegetables

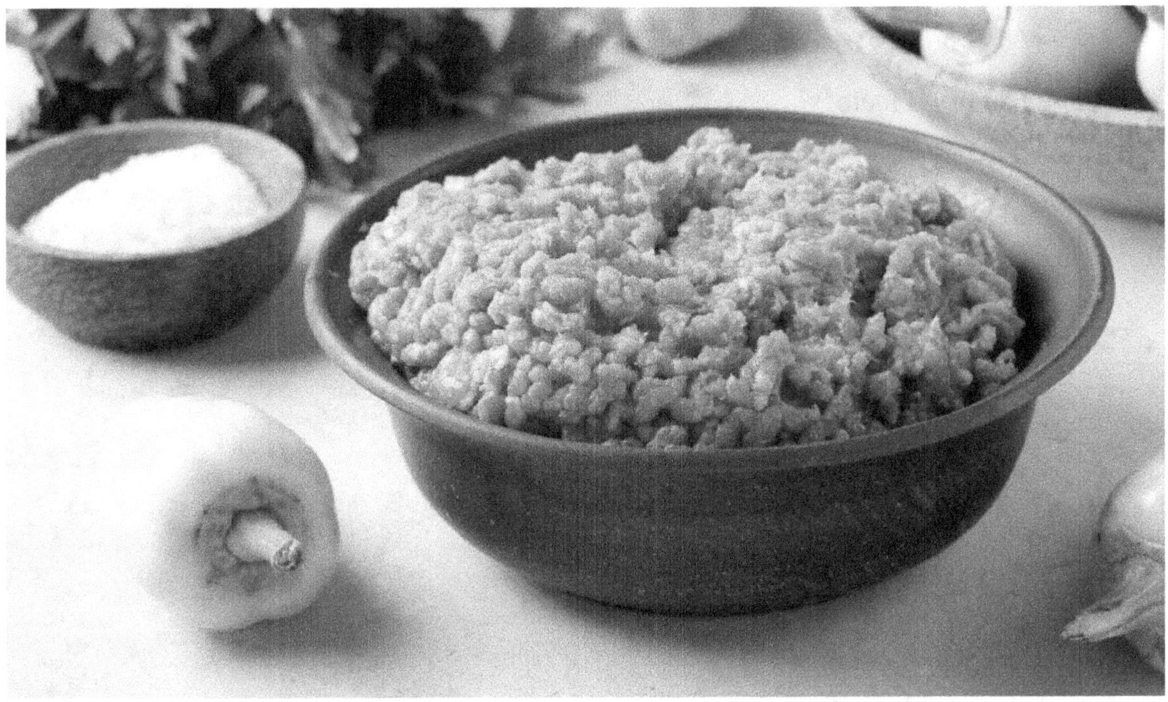

This dish offers a balanced blend of fiber, antioxidants, and lean protein, making it a satisfying and healthy choice for any meal. Enjoy a symphony of flavors and nutrients in every mouthful!

Cooking time: 35 minutes

Servings: 4

Ingredients:

- 1lb lean minced steak
- 7oz courgettes (zucchini), roughly chopped
- 7oz cherry tomatoes
- 4 sprigs of rosemary
- 2 red peppers (bell peppers), roughly chopped
- 2 garlic cloves, crushed
- 2 teaspoons paprika powder
- 1 teaspoon onion powder
- 1 onion, chopped
- 1 butternut squash, peeled, deseeded and chopped
- 1 handful of fresh basil leaves
- 2 tablespoons olive oil
- Sea salt
- Freshly ground black pepper

Instructions:

Place the minced steak into a large bowl, add in the paprika and onion powder and mix well. Season with salt and pepper.

Using clean hands, shape the meat into balls. Place the vegetables, garlic and basil into a large ovenproof dish or baking tray and drizzle olive oil over the top.

Season with salt and pepper and lay the rosemary on top. Make spaces for the meatballs and add them.

Cook in an oven, preheated to 200C/400F for around 25 minutes or until the meatballs are completely cooked. Serve and eat straight away.

28. Lamb & Mint Quinoa

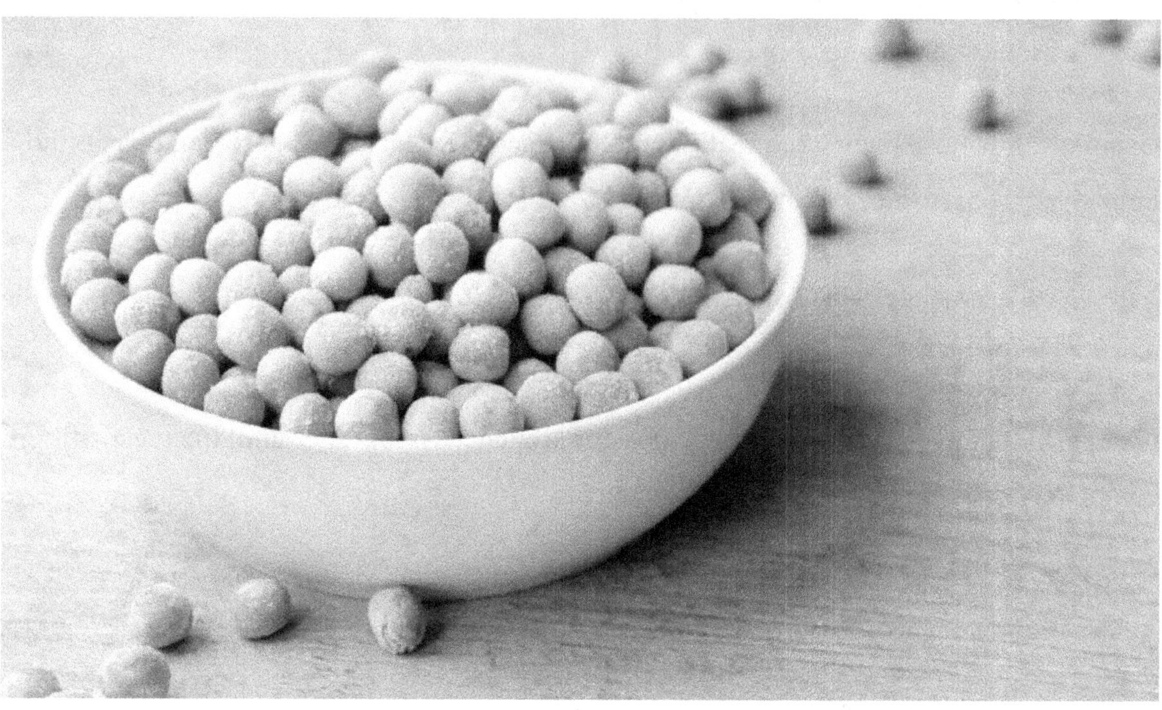

Lean lamb pairs harmoniously with quinoa's nutty goodness, offering a hearty meal that's also heart-healthy. Mint lends a refreshing twist, while adding antioxidants and aiding digestion.

Cooking time: 30 minutes

Servings: 4

Ingredients:

- 1 lb. lean lamb steaks
- 8 oz asparagus, roughly chopped
- 8 oz frozen peas
- 7 oz mange tout (snow peas)
- 5 oz quinoa
- 2 tablespoons fresh mint, roughly chopped
- 1 garlic clove, crushed
- Juice of 1 lemon
- 1 tablespoon olive oil
- 2 teaspoons olive oil
- Chopped mint for garnish

Instructions:

In a bowl, combine a teaspoon of olive oil, lemon juice and garlic in a bowl. Add the lamb, coat it in the mixture and marinate it for around 30 minutes.

In the meantime, cook the quinoa according to the instructions, usually for around 15-20 minutes, until fluffy. Add the mint to the quinoa and stir.

Heat a teaspoon of oil in a frying pan; add the lamb and cook for 9-10 minutes or until it's done to your liking.

While the lamb is cooking, steam the asparagus, peas and mangetout (snow peas) for around 4 minutes until they are tender.

Place the vegetables into a bowl and stir in the lemon juice, garlic and a tablespoon of olive oil and a few chopped mint leaves. Add in the quinoa and mix well.

Serve the quinoa salad with the lamb on top.

29. Slow-Cooked Barbecued Beef

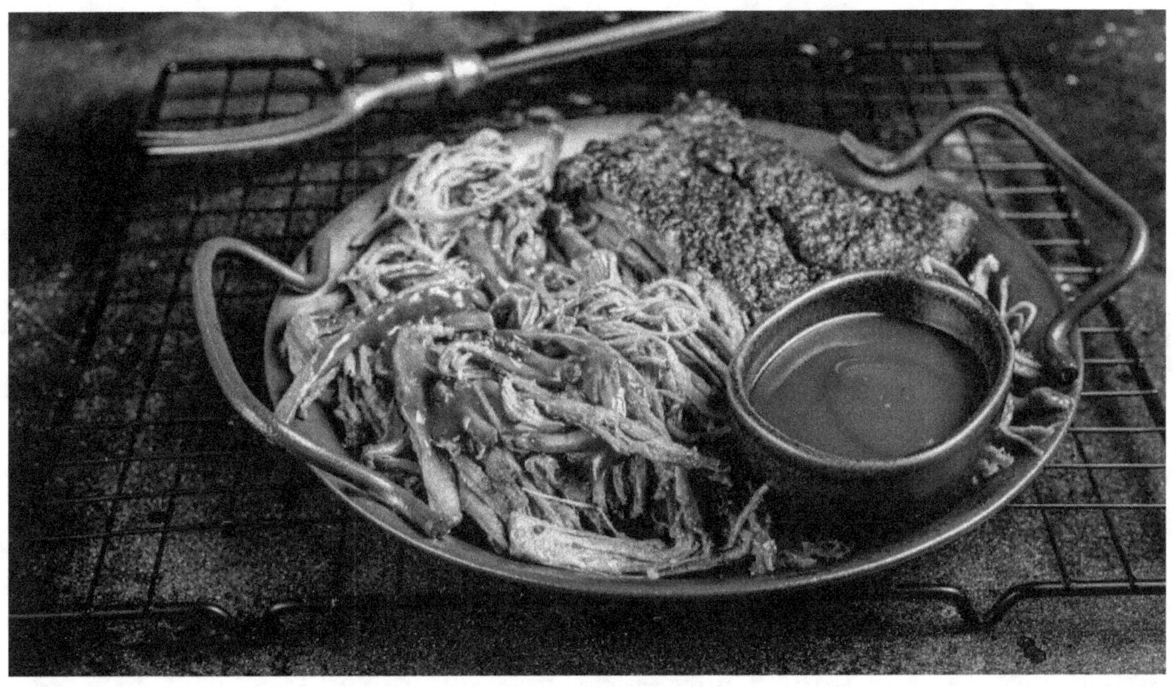

Packed with protein, iron, and zinc, this recipe is a nutrient powerhouse. The slow-cooking process infuses the meat with deep, complex flavors, making each bite a mouthwatering delight.

Cooking time: 8 hours

Servings: 8

Ingredients:

- 1-1/2 pounds extra-lean ground beef (93% lean)
- 2 tbsp extra-virgin olive oil
- 2 tbsp prepared mustard
- 1 cup low-sodium ketchup
- 1 small green bell pepper, chopped
- 3 tbsp vinegar
- 1/2 tsp ground garlic
- 1 tbsp Worcestershire sauce
- 1 medium onion, chopped
- 1 tsp chili powder

Instructions:

Pour the olive oil into a medium skillet and place over medium heat. Once the oil starts to sizzle, add the onions and beef, then brown the beef.

Pour the rest of the ingredients into a slow cooker. Stir.

Add the beef and onions. Stir. Cook on high for 3-4 hours or low for 6-8 hours.

Serve as burgers or sandwiches.

30. Beef and Mushroom Stew

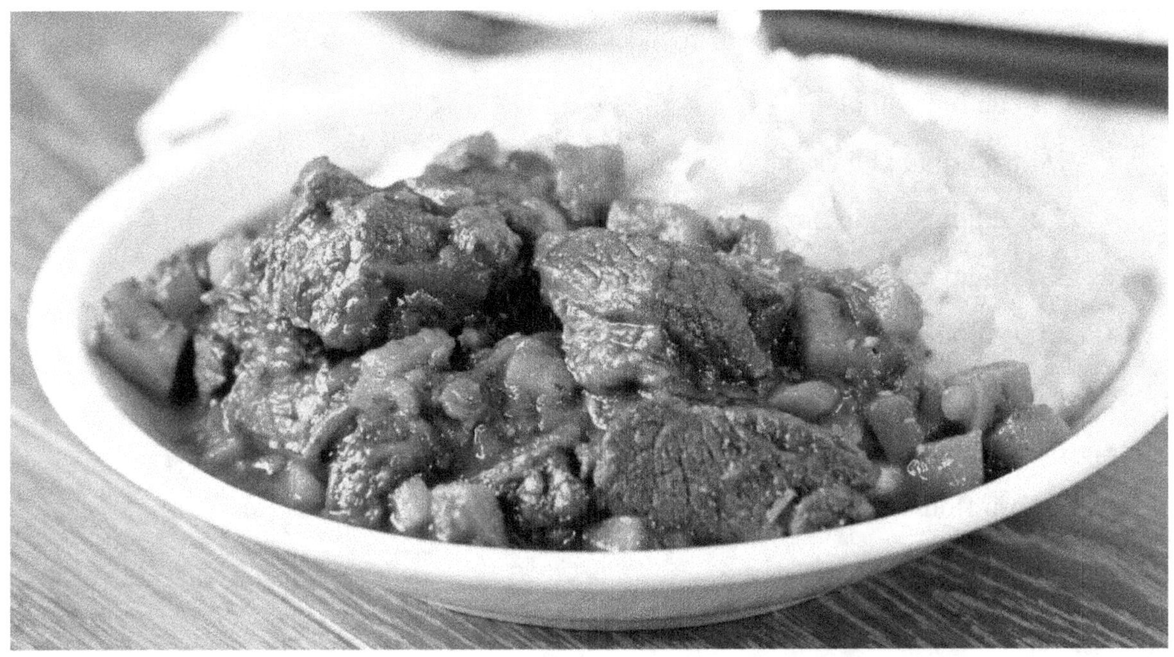

Low in fat and calories, it's a wholesome choice for a balanced diet. This stew, brimming with flavor and nutrients, is comfort in a bowl – perfect for nourishing both body and soul.

Cooking time: 1 hour 5 minutes

Servings: 6

Ingredients:

- 2 cups canned no-salt-added tomatoes
- 14 oz beef broth
- 1/2 cup red wine
- 1/4 tsp ground black pepper
- 5 medium potatoes, quartered
- 3 medium carrots, sliced
- 2 mushrooms, sliced
- 1 bay leaf
- 1/4 tsp dried rosemary
- 3 Tbsp flour
- 1/4 cup of water
- 1-1/2 pounds beef round steak, cut into cubes

Instructions:

Mix all the ingredients (except flour, tomatoes and water) in a large pot and place over medium heat. Cover and cook for 1 hour.

Mix the flour, water and tomatoes in a small bowl.

Add tomato mixture to the pot. Cook until the stew starts to thicken. This may take about 10-20 minutes

Serve and enjoy.

31. Lemon Pork Loin & Roast Winter Vegetables

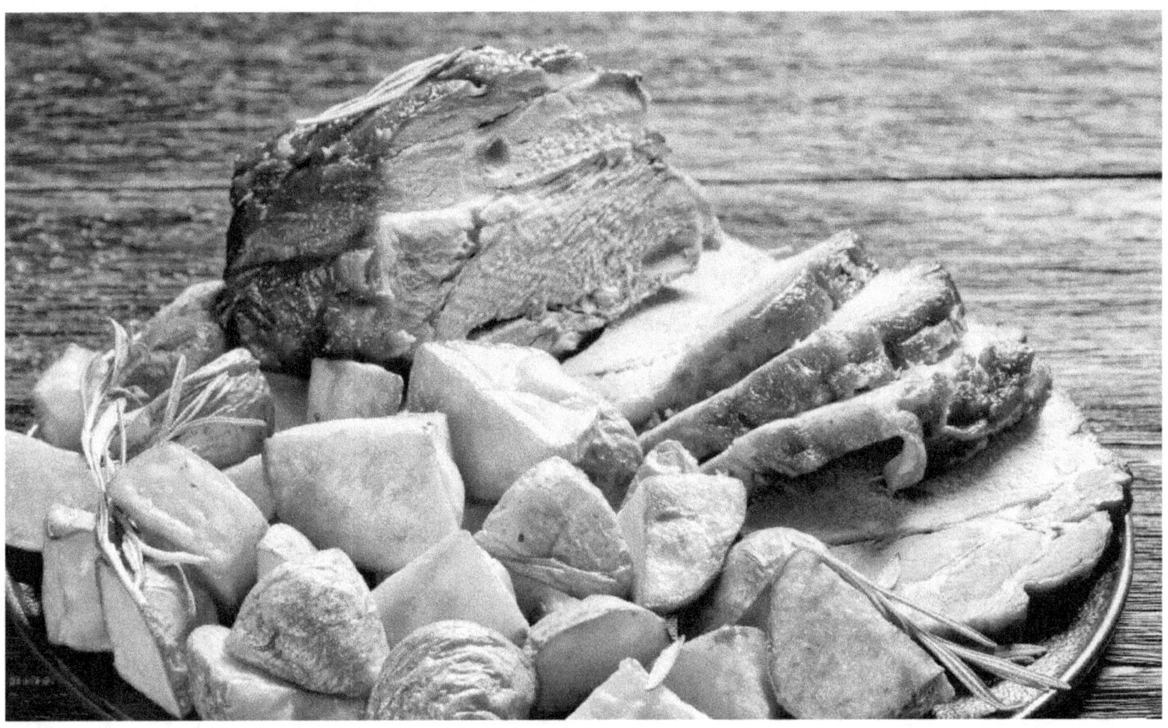

A winter culinary masterpiece that's hearty, wholesome, and guaranteed to tantalize your taste buds.

Cooking time: 30 minutes

Servings: 5

Ingredients:

- 2 lb. boneless pork loin, fat removed where possible
- 1¾lb potatoes, peeled and quartered
- 3 parsnips, peeled roughly chopped
- 2 teaspoons dried mixed herbs
- 2 leeks, roughly chopped
- 1 medium butternut squash, peeled and roughly chopped
- 1 onion, cut into wedges
- 1 teaspoon mustard
- 1 tablespoon vegetable oil
- 1 tablespoon water
- Salt and freshly ground black pepper
- A handful of fresh thyme leaves, roughly chopped
- Juice and zest of 1 lemon

Instructions:

Preheat your oven to 190°C/380F. In a bowl, combine the water, mustard, lemon juice and lemon zest. Place the pork into a roasting tin and spread the mustard marinade over the pork, covering it completely.

Take another roasting tin and scatter the leeks, potatoes, onion, parsnips and squash into the tin. Drizzle the vegetable oil over the top and sprinkle on the dried herbs.

Place the pork into the oven and cook for around 1 hour, or until cooked through. You can test it with a skewer to see if it's done. Remove the pork and let it rest.

Let the vegetables continue cooking for another 10 minutes. Scatter the fresh thyme through the vegetables. Season with salt and pepper.

Slice the pork and serve it alongside the roast veggies. Enjoy.

32. Lamb & Red Pepper Skewers

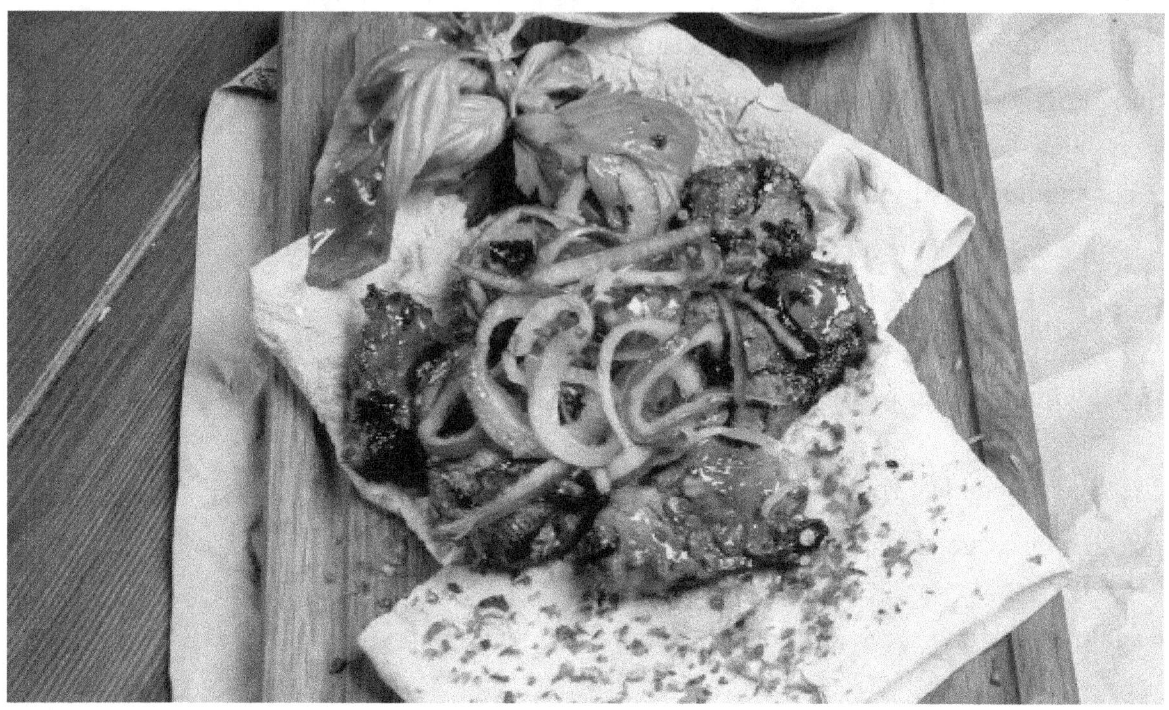

Perfect for summer barbecues or quick weeknight dinners, these skewers are a savory delight that satisfies every palate.

Cooking time: 15 minutes

Servings: 2

Ingredients:

- 9 oz lean lamb steaks, cut into bite-sized chunks
- 1 tablespoon tomato purée (paste)
- 3 cloves of garlic, crushed
- 1 red pepper (bell pepper), cut into chunks
- 1 small red onion, cut into chunks
- ½ teaspoon onion powder
- 1 teaspoon smoked paprika
- 1 tablespoon olive oil

Instructions:

Place the paprika, tomato purée (paste), onion powder, garlic and olive oil into a bowl and mix well.

Add the lamb chunks and coat them well in the marinade. Cover them and let it marinate for at least an hour.

Thread the meat, onion and pepper onto skewers, alternating the ingredients.

Place the skewers under a preheated grill (broiler) and cook for 9-10 minutes, turning during cooking until the lamb is cooked through.

Chapter 5: Salads and Soups Recipes

33. Watermelon & Arugula Salad

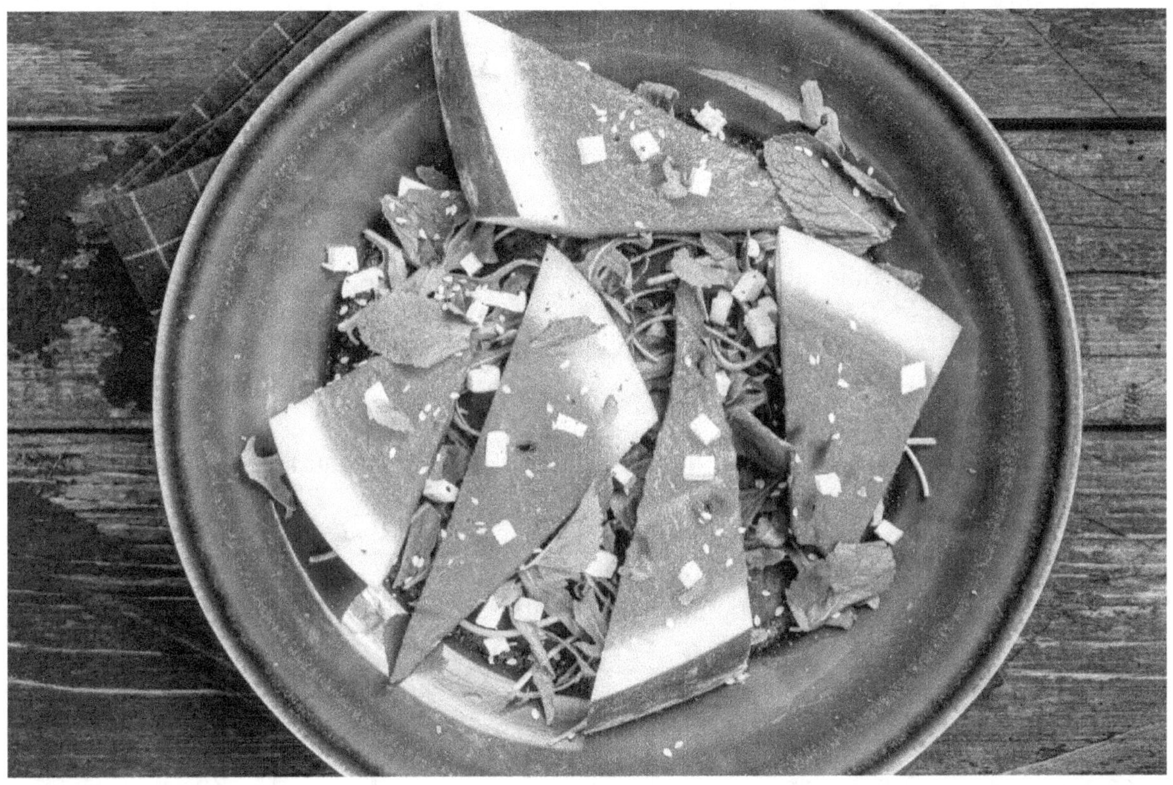

This salad is a harmonious blend of sweetness, peppery notes, and savory goodness. It's a light and vibrant addition to any meal or a standalone treat that celebrates the essence of summer on your plate.

Cooking time: 5 minutes

Servings: 4

Ingredients:

- 4 cups cubed watermelon
- 2 cups arugula
- 1 cup diced cucumber
- ¼ teaspoon salt
- 2 tablespoons pumpkin seeds
- ¼ cup Classic Balsamic Vinaigrette

Instructions:

In a large bowl, gently toss together the watermelon, arugula, cucumber, and salt until well mixed.

Just before serving, top with the pumpkin seeds and vinaigrette.

34. Fresh Cucumber & Avocado Salad

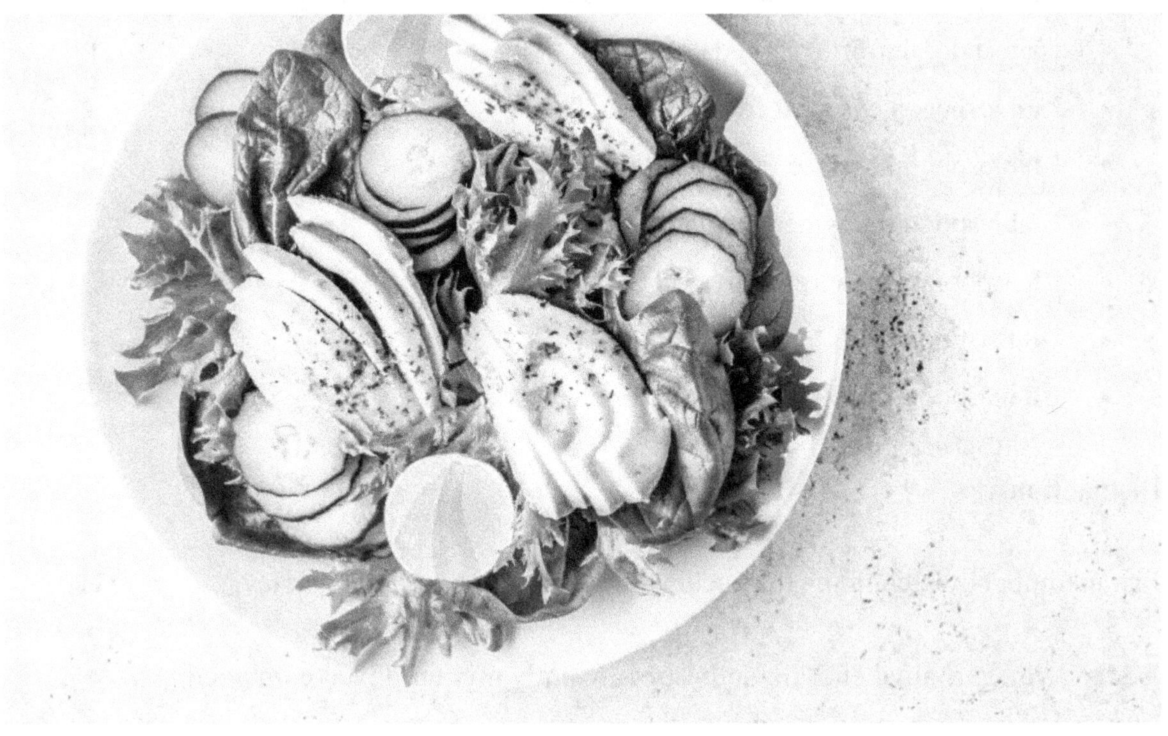

It's a delightful blend of freshness and zest that will invigorate your taste buds and nourish your body.

Cooking time: 20 minutes

Servings: 4

Ingredients:

- 2 medium cucumbers, uniformly diced
- 1 avocado, uniformly diced
- 2 tablespoons chopped fresh basil
- 1 tablespoon chopped fresh parsley
- 1 tablespoon red wine vinegar
- 1 teaspoon extra-virgin olive oil
- 1/8 teaspoon salt
- 1/8 teaspoon freshly ground black pepper

Instructions:

In a medium bowl, combine the cucumbers, avocado, basil, and parsley.

Add the vinegar, olive oil, salt, and pepper. Gently mix until well combined.

Refrigerate to marinate for 15 minutes. Stir again just before serving.

35. Lemon Kale Chopped Salad

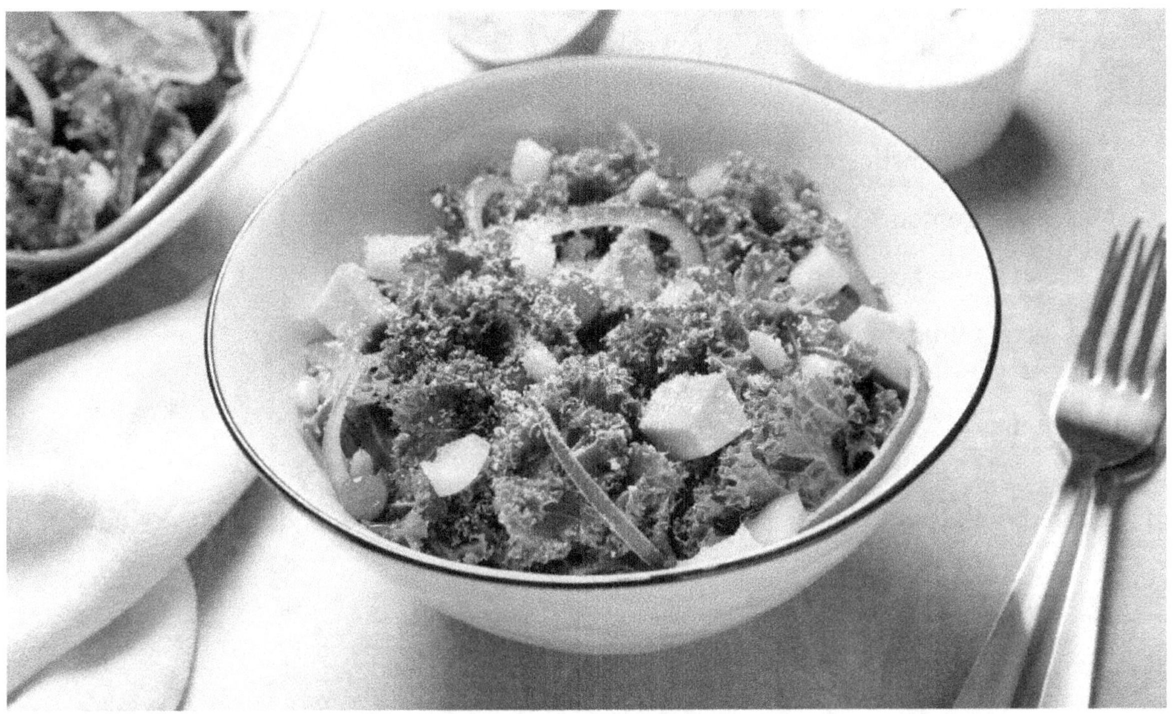

Lemon Kale Chopped Salad is a refreshing, nutrient-packed dish. This salad is a symphony of textures and tastes, perfect for a quick, healthy meal.

Cooking time: 15 minutes

Servings: 4

Ingredients:

- 2 cups chopped kale
- 1 cup chopped radicchio, or red cabbage
- 1 cup shredded Brussels sprouts
- ½ cup matchstick carrots
- ½ cup Lemon Vinaigrette
- ¼ cup dried cranberries
- ¼ cup pumpkin seeds

Instructions:

In a large bowl, toss together the kale, radicchio, Brussels sprouts, and carrots until well mixed.

Pour in the vinaigrette and toss until everything is well coated.

Just before serving, top the salad with the cranberries and pumpkin seeds.

36. Mushroom Soup

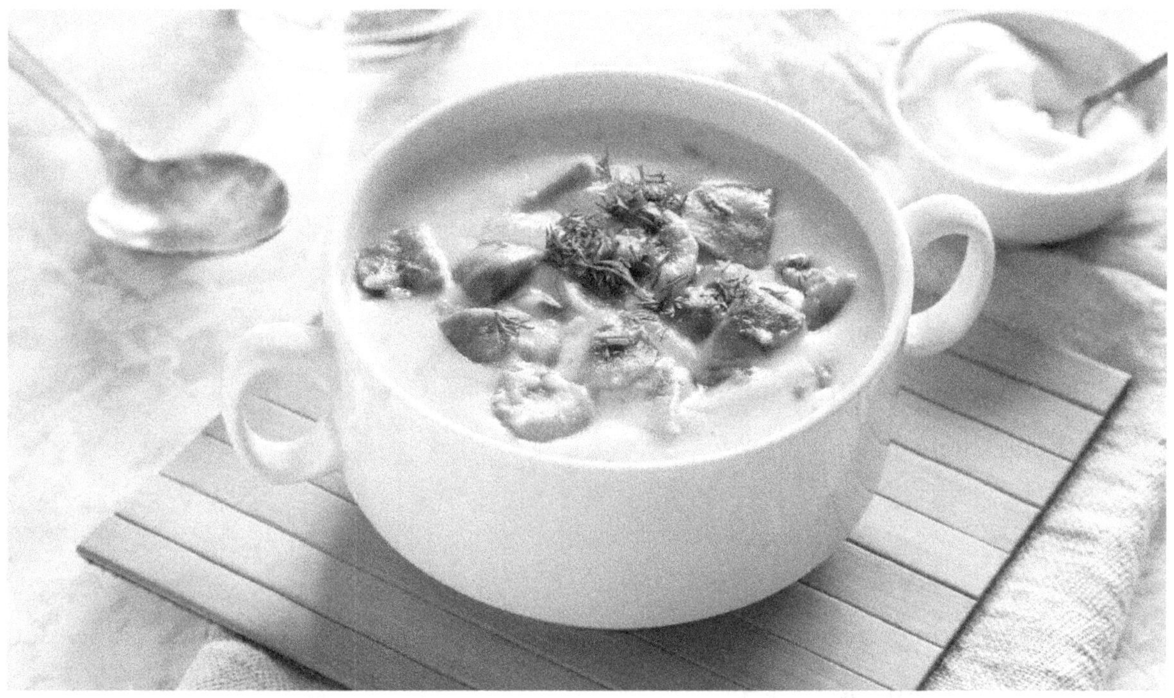

Crafted from a medley of fresh mushrooms, sautéed to perfection, this soup delivers a velvety, umami-packed experience.

Cooking time: 35 minutes

Servings: 6

Ingredients:

- 2 medium onions, finely chopped
- 2 tablespoons sunflower oil
- 2 pounds mushrooms, finely chopped
- 2 gluten free vegetable stock cubes
- Salt to taste
- Pepper to taste
- Handful fresh parsley, chopped
- 6 teaspoons corn flour mixed with 2 tablespoons water
- 1 cup single cream

Instructions:

Place a large soup pot over medium heat. Add oil. When the oil is heated, add onions and sauté until golden brown.

Stir in the mushrooms and cook for 4-5 minutes. Stir constantly.

Boil 5 cups of water and add stock cubes into it. Let it dissolve.

Pour stock into the soup pot. Add parsley, salt and pepper and bring to the boil.

Lower heat and cover with a lid. Simmer for 15-20 minutes.

Add corn flour mixture and stir constantly until thick.

Add cream and stir.

Ladle into soup bowls and serve.

37. Turkey and Vegetable Soup in Coconut Curry

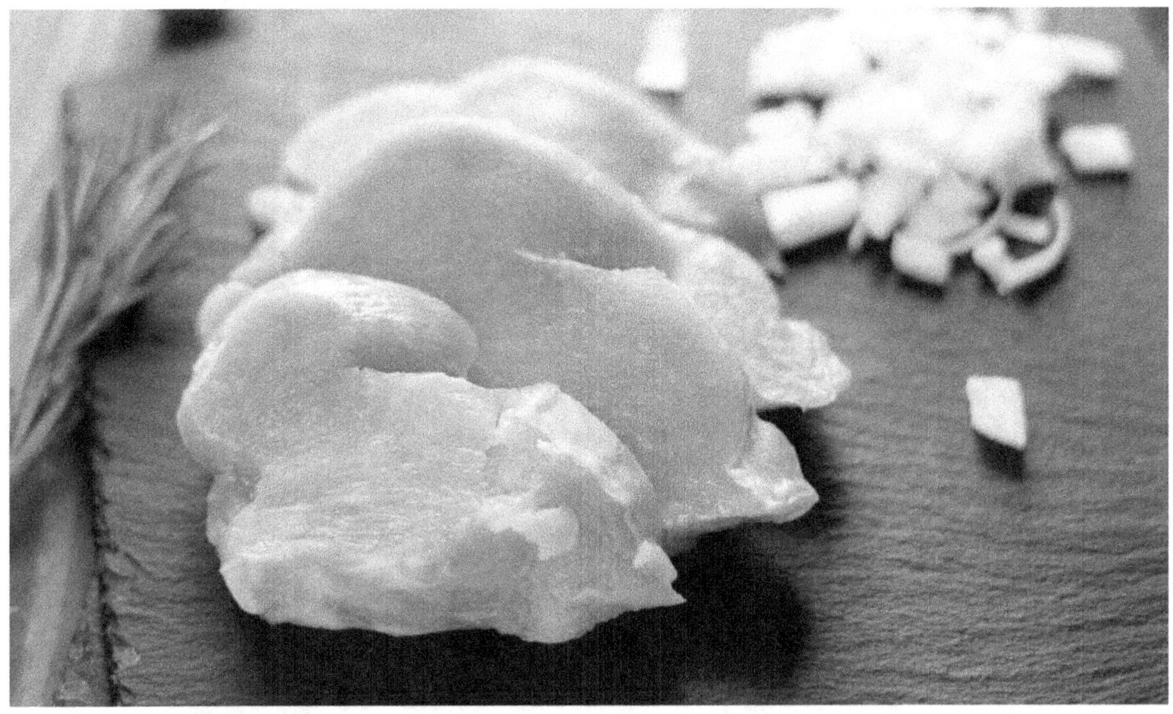

Warm the belly with this creamy coconut curry soup! This is a great thyroid-friendly dish if there is leftover turkey in the refrigerator, but chicken could be used, too. This soup can be made pretty quickly. I'm a fan of frozen green beans and broccoli when making soup for convenience, but fresh vegetables are always welcome.

Cooking time: 35 minutes

Servings: 6

Ingredients:

- 2 (14-ounce) cans light coconut milk
- 2 cups Chicken Bone Broth
- 2 teaspoons Ginger-Turmeric Rub
- 2 teaspoons red curry powder
- 1 garlic clove, minced
- 2 cups cooked turkey, cut into 1-inch chunks
- 2 cups broccoli, coarsely chopped
- 1 cup frozen green beans
- 1 red bell pepper, chopped
- ½ cup fresh cilantro, chopped (optional)

Instructions:

In a large soup pot, combine the coconut milk, broth, ginger-turmeric rub, red curry powder, and garlic. Cook over medium heat for 10 minutes.

Add the turkey, broccoli, green beans, and red bell pepper. Cook for 10 to 15 minutes, or until the vegetables are soft. Remove from the heat.

Serve the soup hot, garnished with the cilantro (if using).

38. Summer Squash & Carrot Soup

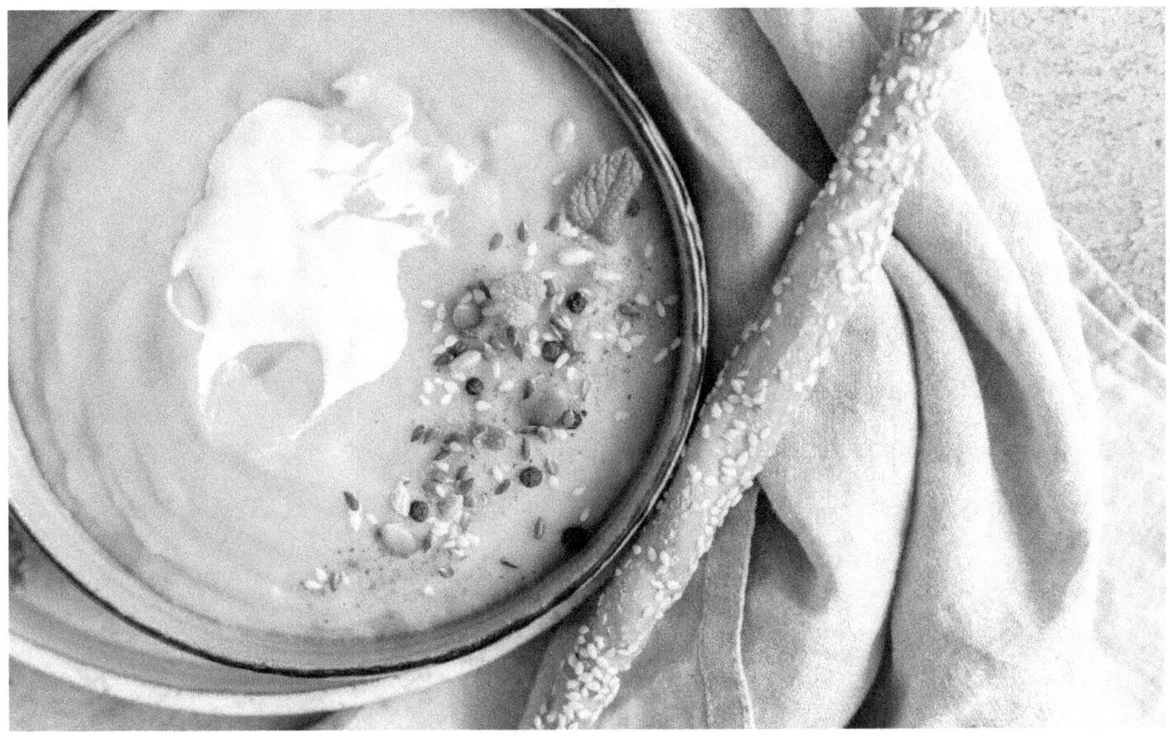

This vibrant, velvety concoction combines tender summer squash and sweet carrots, creating a harmonious blend that's both nutritious and satisfying.

Cooking time: 30 minutes

Servings: 4

Ingredients:

- 5 cups diced seeded summer squash, divided
- 3 cups chopped carrot
- 6 cups vegetable stock, or Chicken Bone Broth
- 2 tablespoons extra-virgin olive oil
- 1 cup diced Spanish onion
- 2 tablespoons chopped shallot
- 1 tablespoon chopped garlic
- ½ bunch fresh parsley, chopped
- 2 teaspoons ground ginger
- 1 teaspoon salt
- ½ teaspoon freshly ground black pepper

Instructions:

In a small soup pot over medium-high heat, combine half the squash and all the carrots. Cover the vegetables with the vegetable stock. Cook for about 5 minutes, or until very tender.

In a large stockpot over medium-low heat, heat the olive oil. Add the onion, shallot, and garlic. Sweat until aromatic, 3 to 4 minutes.

Add the remaining squash to the stockpot. Continue cooking for about 5 minutes, or until almost tender.

When the carrots and squash are tender, using an immersion blender, blend until smooth. Alternatively, transfer the contents to a traditional blender (you may have to work in batches) and purée until smooth. Pour the puréed carrot mixture into the stockpot. Stir to combine.

Add the parsley, ginger, salt, and pepper. Cook on low heat for 5 minutes until combined and warmed through.

39. Hearty Beef & Vegetable Soup

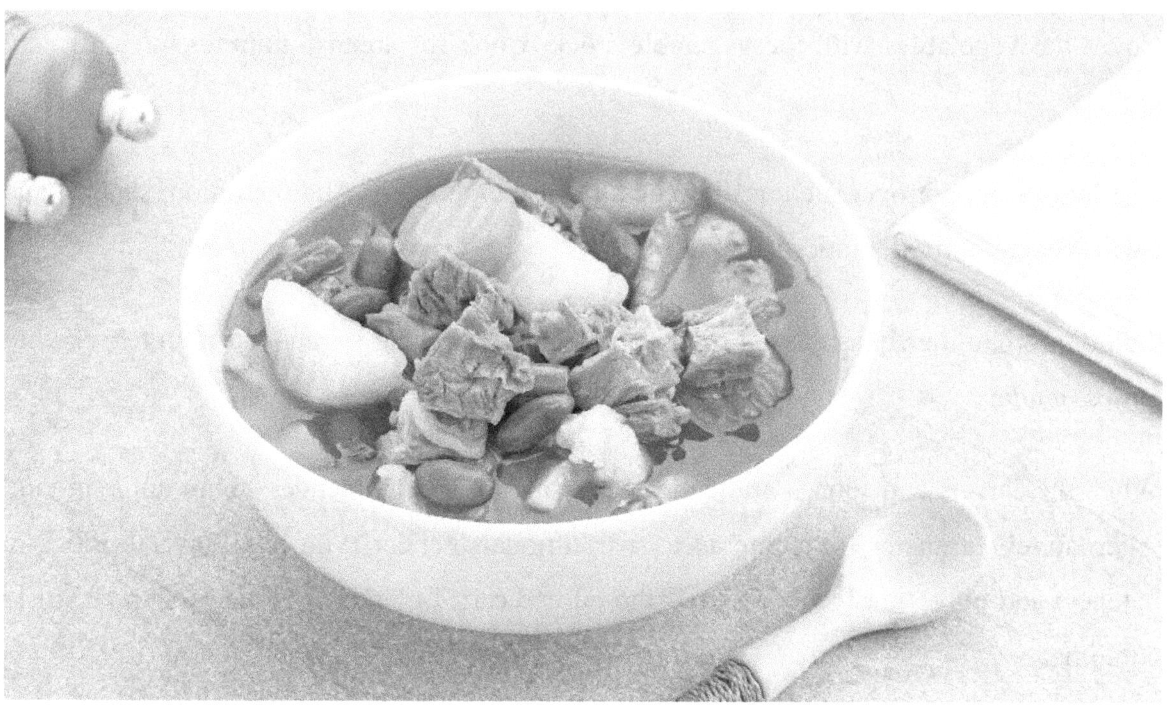

This wonderful soup brings together the nutritious benefits of vegetables, lean protein, and bone broth for a comforting, nourishing bowl of goodness that's delicious any time of day.

Cooking time: 30 minutes

Servings: 4

Ingredients:

- 2 tablespoons extra-virgin olive oil, divided
- 1 pound beef stew meat, cut into 1-inch chunks
- 1 teaspoon salt, divided
- 1 teaspoon freshly ground black pepper, divided
- 1 cup diced white onion
- 1 cup diced carrot
- 1 cup diced celery
- 2 cups diced sweet potato
- 1 tablespoon minced garlic
- 6 cups Slow Cooker Savory Beef Bone Broth
- 2 bay leaves
- 2 cups chopped kale
- 1 tablespoon chopped fresh parsley, for garnish

Instructions:

In a large soup pot over medium heat, heat 1 tablespoon of olive oil.

Season the stew meat with ½ teaspoon of salt and ½ teaspoon of pepper. Add the beef to the pot. Cook for 4 to 5 minutes until browned. Remove from the pot and set aside.

Add the remaining 1 tablespoon of olive oil to the pot along with the onion, carrot, celery, sweet potato, and garlic. Sauté for 5 minutes, stirring frequently.

Return the meat to the pot. Add the beef broth, bay leaves, and remaining ½ teaspoon each of salt and pepper. Bring the soup to a boil. Reduce the heat to a simmer and cook for 15 minutes.

Stir in the kale. Simmer for 2 minutes more.

Remove and discard the bay leaves. Just before serving, garnish the stew with the parsley.

40. Chipotle Pumpkin Soup

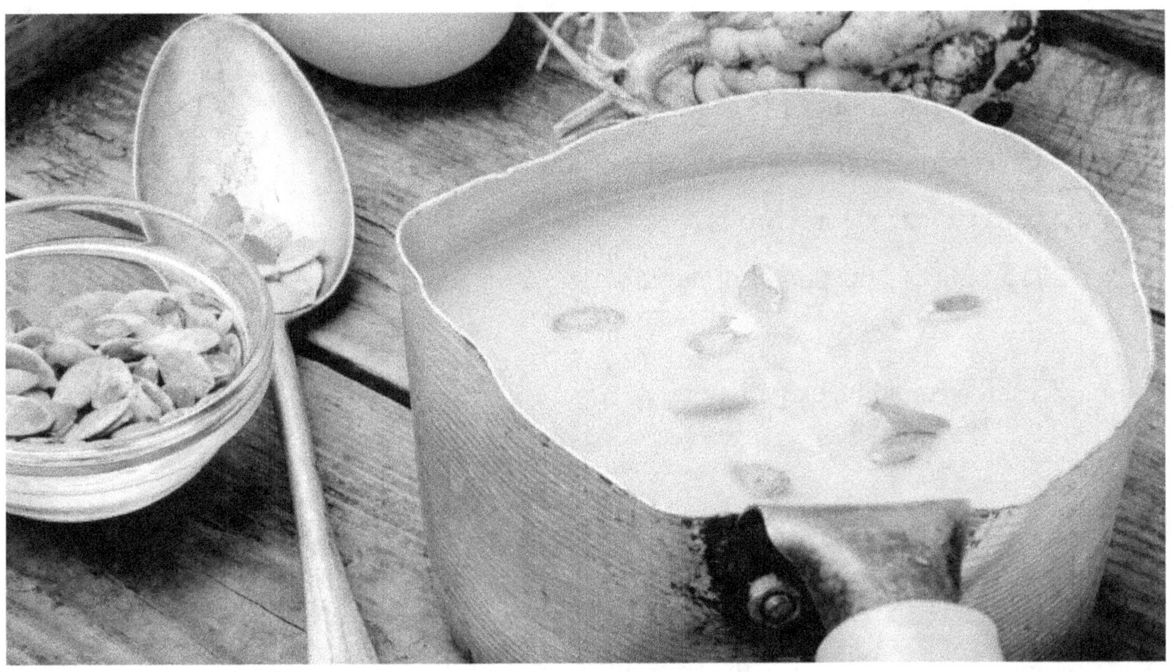

This is one of my favorite soups to make in a pinch and is especially delicious in colder months. Pumpkin combined with chicken bone broth gives the soup a delicious, creamy texture. This recipe is high in beta-carotene and vitamin C, two important antioxidants that fight inflammation associated with thyroid disease.

Cooking time: 35 minutes

Servings: 4

Ingredients:

- 1 tablespoon extra-virgin olive oil
- 1 large onion, diced
- 1 garlic clove, minced
- 1 tablespoon ground chipotle pepper
- 4 cups Chicken Bone Broth
- 2 (15-ounce) cans pumpkin puree
- Salt
- Freshly ground black pepper

Instructions:

In a large soup pot or Dutch oven, heat the oil over medium heat.

Add the onion and garlic. Cook for 5 minutes, or until the onion is translucent.

Add the chipotle pepper and toss the onion and garlic to coat.

Add the broth and pumpkin puree. Stir to combine.

Reduce the heat to medium-low. Simmer for 20 to 25 minutes. Season with salt and pepper. Remove from the heat.

41. Brussels Sprout Salad

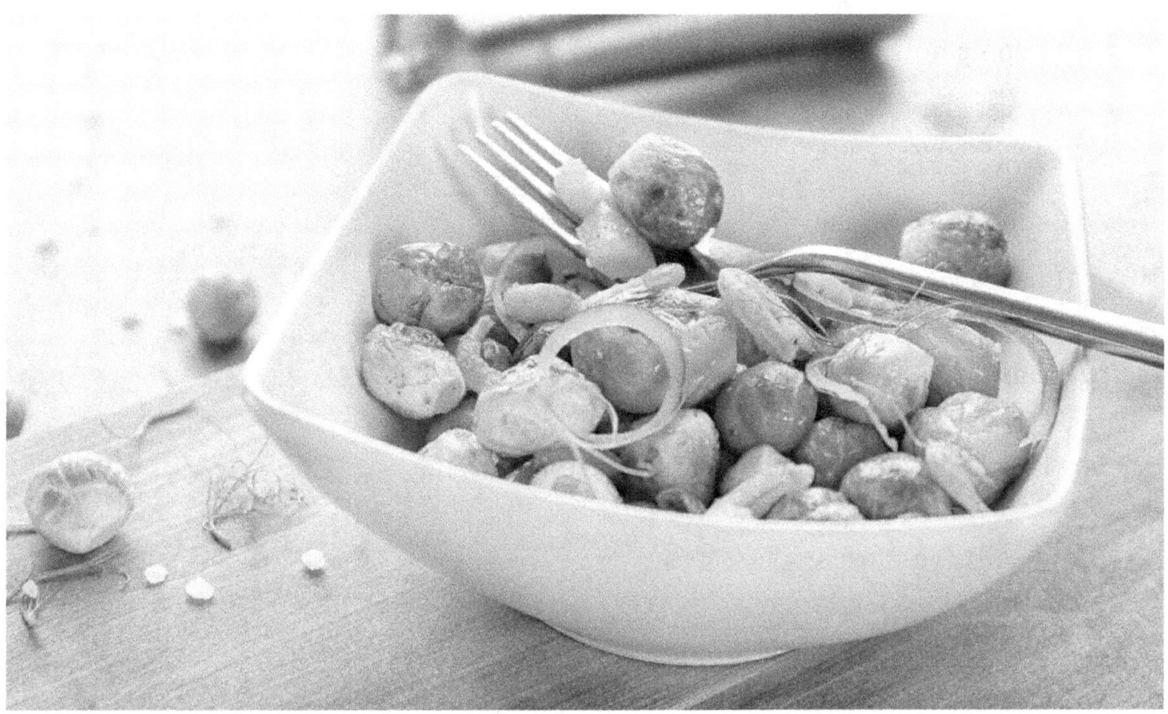

This salad, a blend of freshness and depth, makes a perfect side or a light, satisfying meal. It's a testament to how simple ingredients can create a culinary masterpiece.

Cooking time: 10 minutes

Servings: 2

Ingredients:

- 1 tablespoon olive oil
- 1 cup shallots
- ½ cup celery
- 1 clove garlic
- 6-8 brussels sprouts
- 1 tablespoon thyme leaves

Instructions:

In a bowl, combine all ingredients together and mix well.

Serve with dressing.

42. Meatball Soup

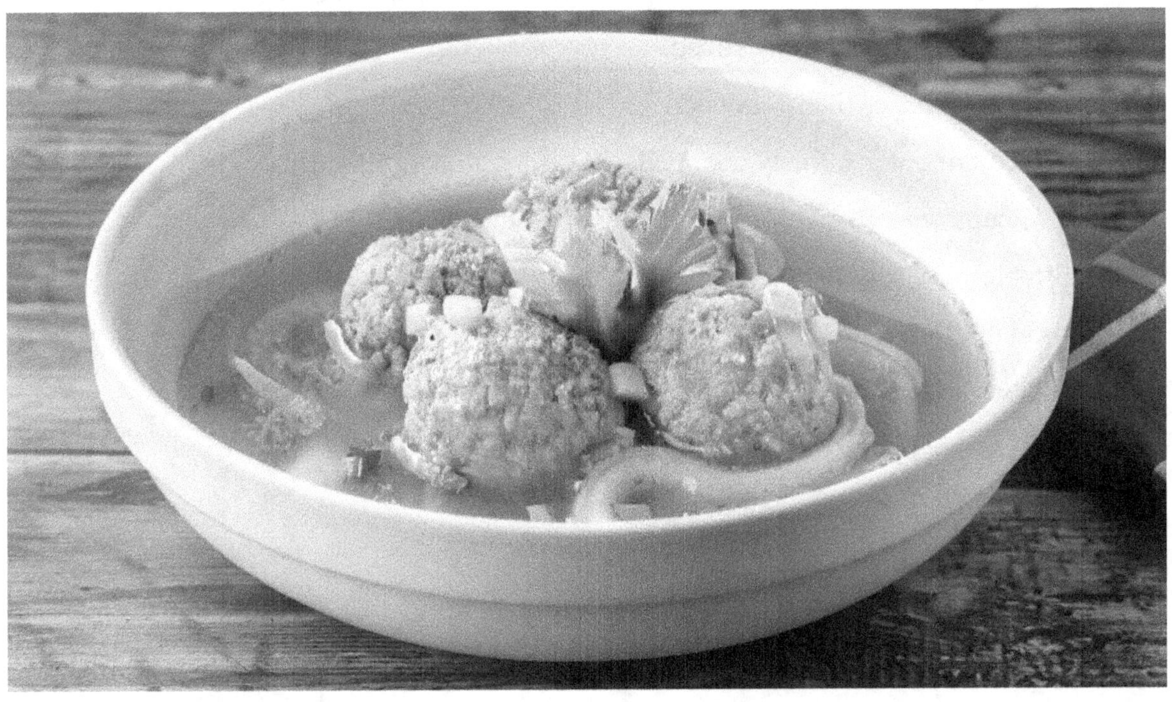

A hearty and comforting dish, combines succulent meatballs with a flavorful broth and an array of vegetables.

Cooking time: 35 minutes

Servings: 8

Ingredients:

- 21 ounces minced or ground pork or beef or a mixture of both
- 2 medium carrots, thinly sliced
- 2 cups cabbage, finely chopped
- 2 medium onions, finely chopped
- 1 ½ cups winter squash or courgette, cut into small cubes
- 3 tablespoons garlic, chopped
- 4-5 tablespoons homemade sauerkraut
- Salt to taste
- Cayenne pepper to taste
- Fresh dill, finely chopped to garnish
- Yogurt to garnish

Instructions:

Add ground meat into a bowl. Make small balls of the mixture of about ¾ inch diameter.

Place a soup pot over medium heat. Add about 8-10 cups water. Bring to the boil.

Add salt and cayenne pepper and stir.

Drop the meatballs in the water. Drop one at a time.

Lower heat to low. Cover with a lid. Simmer for around 30 minutes.

Add carrot, cabbage, onions and winter squash.

Cover the lid and simmer until vegetables are tender.

Add garlic and stir. Turn off heat. Let it cover and sit for a while.

Add sauerkraut and stir.

Ladle into soup bowls and serve garnished with dill and yogurt.

43. Arugula Salad with Salmon, Avocado and Tomato

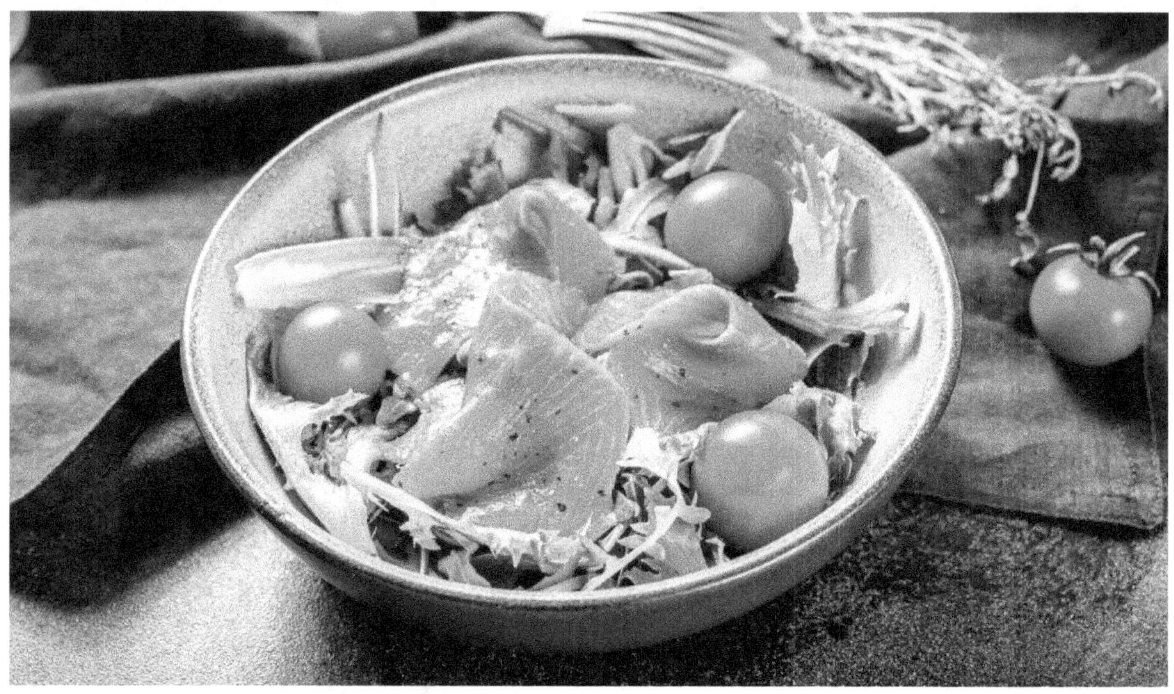

This salad is a healthy, flavorful masterpiece that's quick and easy to prepare.

Cooking time: 5 minutes

Servings: 2

Ingredients:

- 1 (10 oz) can salmon, drained, chopped into bite sized pieces
- 3 cups baby arugula
- 1 small avocado, peeled, pitted, sliced
- 2 tablespoons red onion, thinly sliced
- 4 medium radishes, peeled, thinly sliced
- 1 tomato, chopped into chunks

For the dressing:

- Sea salt to taste
- Freshly ground black pepper to taste
- ½ teaspoon honey
- 1 tablespoon extra-virgin olive oil
- 1 tablespoon balsamic vinegar

Instructions:

Place the arugula in a serving bowl. Layer with avocado followed by onion, radish and tomato and finally salmon.

To make the dressing: Whisk together all the ingredients of the dressing in a bowl. Pour over the salad and serve.

Chapter 6: Desserts Recipes

44. Roasted Sweet Potato Wedges

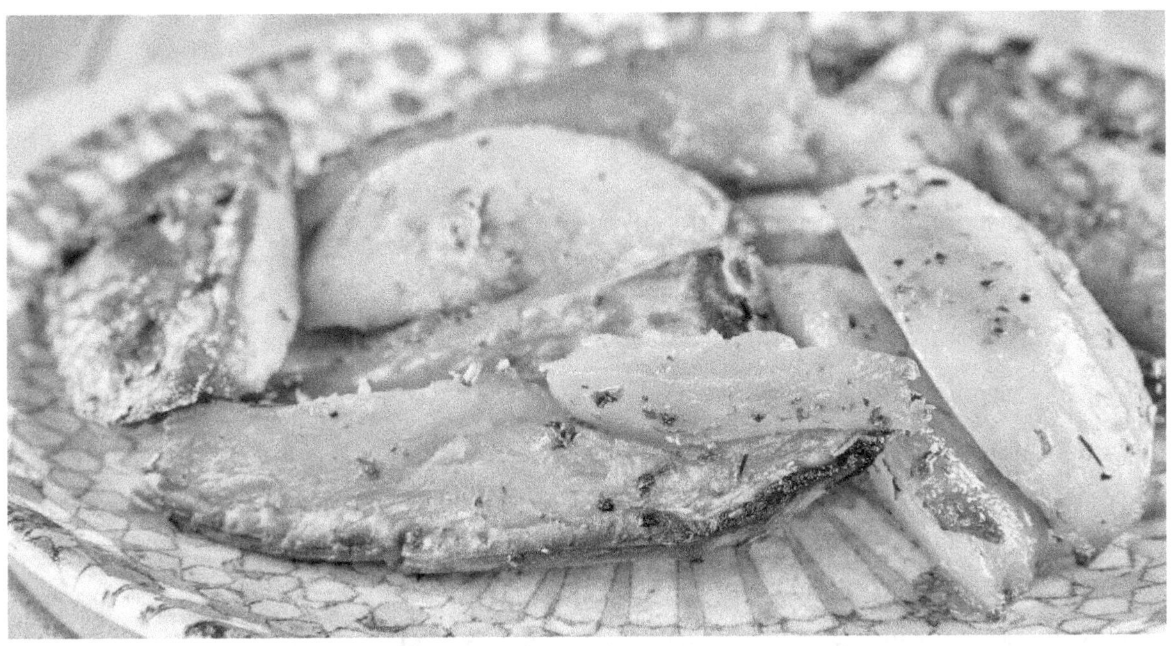

These wedges, tender on the inside and crispy on the outside, offer a sweet and savory symphony of flavors, making them a wholesome side dish or a guilt-free snack.

Cooking time: 30 minutes

Servings: 8

Ingredients:

- 8 medium sweet potatoes, cut into wedges
- Sea salt to taste
- Pepper powder to taste
- Chili flakes to taste
- ½ teaspoon dry tarragon (optional)
- ½ teaspoon dried oregano (optional)
- ½ teaspoon ground cumin (optional)
- ½ teaspoon dried thyme (optional)
- 4 tablespoons coconut oil, melted

Instructions:

Add sweet potatoes into a bowl. Sprinkle oil on it. Toss well.

Sprinkle salt, pepper, chili flakes and any other optional herbs that you are using on it. Toss well.

Place a sheet of parchment paper on a baking sheet.

Spread the sweet potatoes on the baking sheet. Spread it in a single layer and do not overlap.

Bake in a preheated oven at 425° F for about 45 minutes. Turn the sweet potatoes a couple of times while it is baking.

If you leave the door of the oven slightly open, the wedges turn out crisp.

45. Creamy Lime Pudding

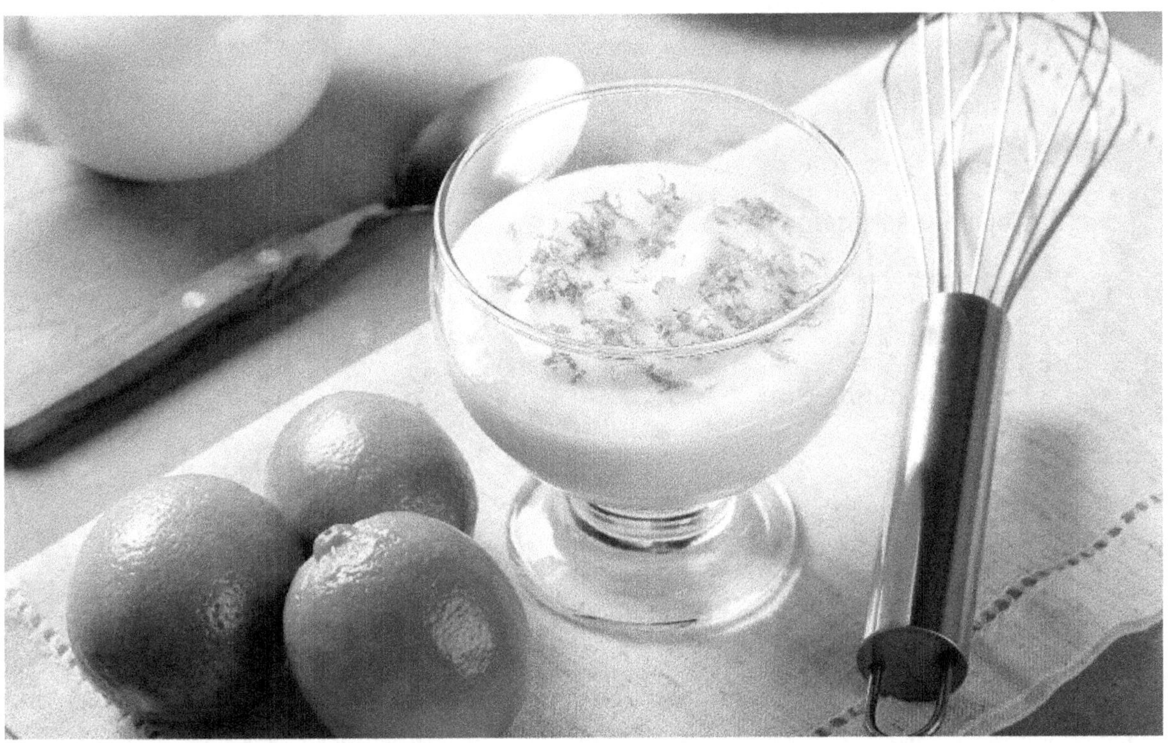

This recipe effortlessly transforms everyday ingredients into a tropical sensation that'll transport your palate to a sunny paradise.

Cooking time: 8 minutes

Servings: 43

Ingredients:

- 4 ounces cashews
- 2 tablespoons coconut butter
- 1 teaspoon lime juice
- ¼ teaspoon rose water
- 3 drops Stevia (optional)
- ½ cup water
- Zest of ½ lime
- ½ teaspoon vanilla extract
- A pinch salt
- Few rose petals to garnish

Instructions:

Add cashews, coconut butter, lime juice, rose water, Stevia, water, lime zest, vanilla and salt into a blender. Blend until smooth.

Divide into serving bowls. Chill for a couple of hours.

Garnish with rose petals and serve.

46. Yogurt Vanilla Smoothie

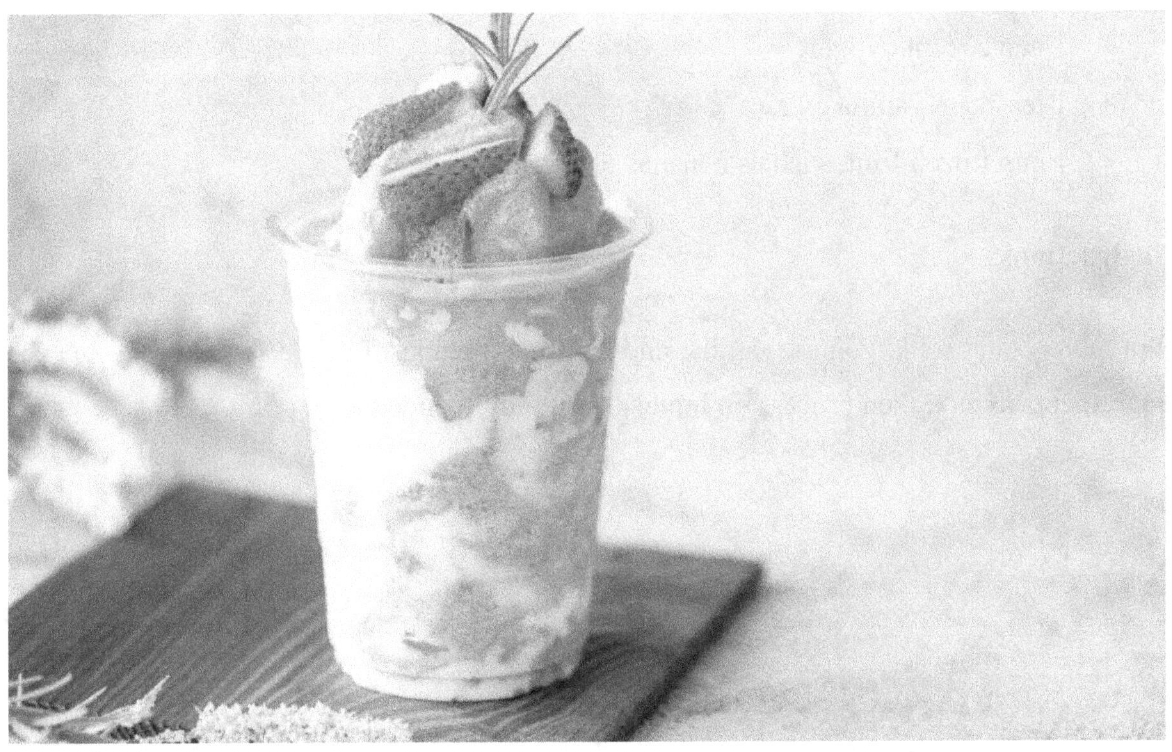

Who doesn't love a nutritious smoothie for breakfast or as a snack? With the right ingredients, loads of nutrition can be added to a diet. To give the smoothie body, this recipe uses creamy, coconut-based yogurt, which is available in most grocery stores. Coconut milk, or a favorite juice, can be used for the liquid, depending on which diet is in play.

Cooking time: 10 minutes

Servings: 2

Ingredients:

- 1 cup coconut milk
- 1 cup coconut yogurt
- 1 teaspoon vanilla extract
- 1 cup frozen fruit, such as bananas or berries

Instructions:

Put the coconut milk, yogurt, vanilla, and fruit in a blender. Pulse a few times to get the ingredients to mix, then process on liquefy until fully blended.

47. Baked Olives

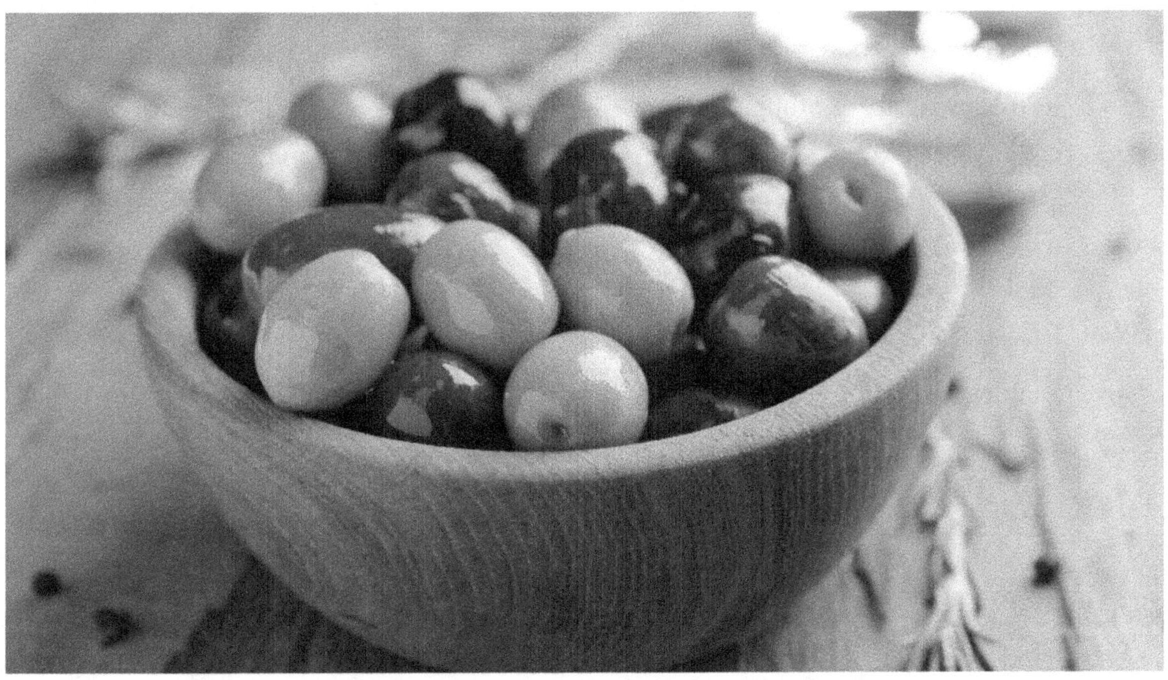

An alluring dish that bursts with briny, earthy, and citrusy notes. Serve them warm, and let your taste buds embark on a delightful Mediterranean journey that's both elegant and easy.

Cooking time: 20 minutes

Servings: 6

Ingredients:

- 9oz whole mixed olives, drained
- 2 tablespoons apple cider vinegar
- 1 tablespoon fresh orange juice
- 1 tablespoon olive oil
- 2 cloves garlic, finely chopped
- 2 sprigs fresh rosemary
- 1 tablespoon fresh parsley, chopped
- 1 tablespoon chopped fresh oregano
- 2 teaspoons grated orange zest
- Pinch of chilli flakes

Instructions:

Preheat the oven to 190C/ 380F.

Place the olives in an ovenproof dish and mix in the vinegar, orange juice, olive oil, rosemary and garlic.

Transfer them to the oven and cook for 15 minutes.

Remove the rosemary and add in the herbs, chilli flakes and orange zest. Can be served warm or cold.

48. Gluten Free Garlic & Herb Crackers

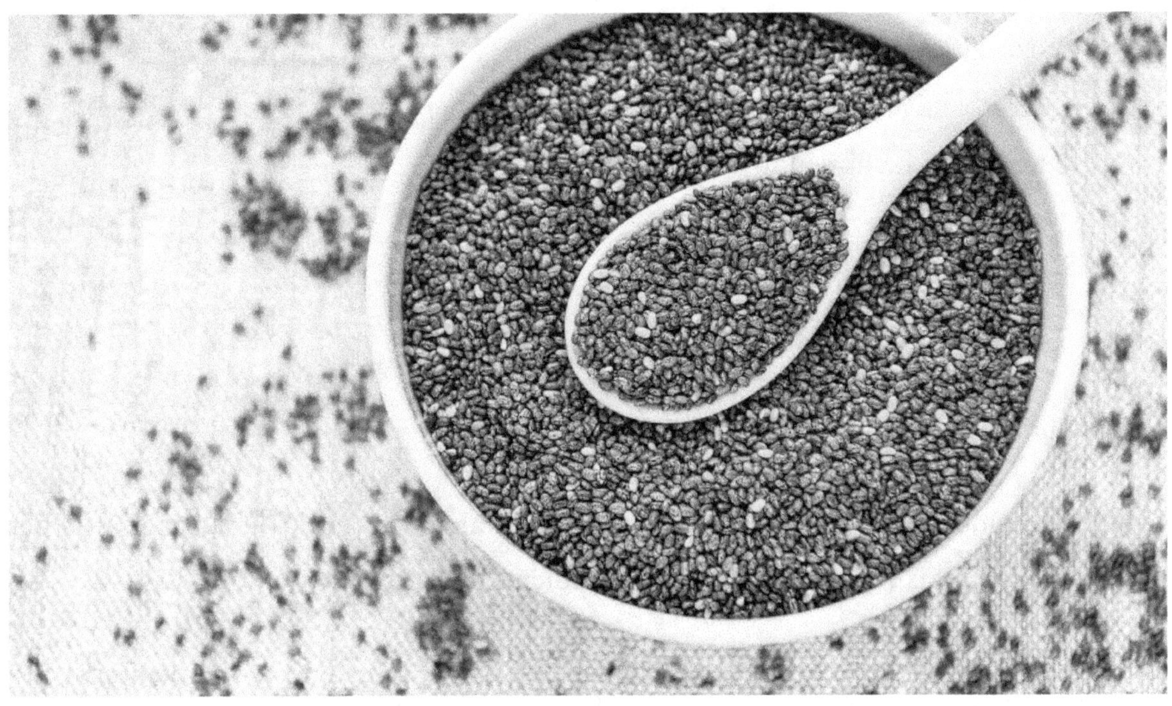

Crafted to perfection, they boast a crisp texture and a rich flavor profile that'll keep you coming back for more. Made without any gluten, they're an excellent choice for those with dietary restrictions.

Cooking time: 55 minutes

Servings: 4

Ingredients:

- 3 oz chia seeds
- 3 oz sunflower seeds
- 2 oz ground almonds (almond meal/almond flour)
- 2 teaspoons herbs de Provence or mixed herbs
- 1 clove of garlic, crushed
- ¼ teaspoon sea salt
- 1 cup cold water

Instructions:

In a bowl, combine the sunflower seeds, chia seeds, almonds, garlic, herbs and salt. Pour in the water and mix really well until the ingredients thicken.

Grease and line a baking tray and spoon the mixture into it, spreading and smoothing it out.

Transfer it to the oven, preheated to 170C/340F and cook for 25 minutes. Remove it and carefully cut it into slices.

Return it to the oven and cook for another 25 minutes. Once cooled, store in an airtight container.

Use as a snack or serve with salads and dips.

49. Avocado and Mango Lettuce Wrap

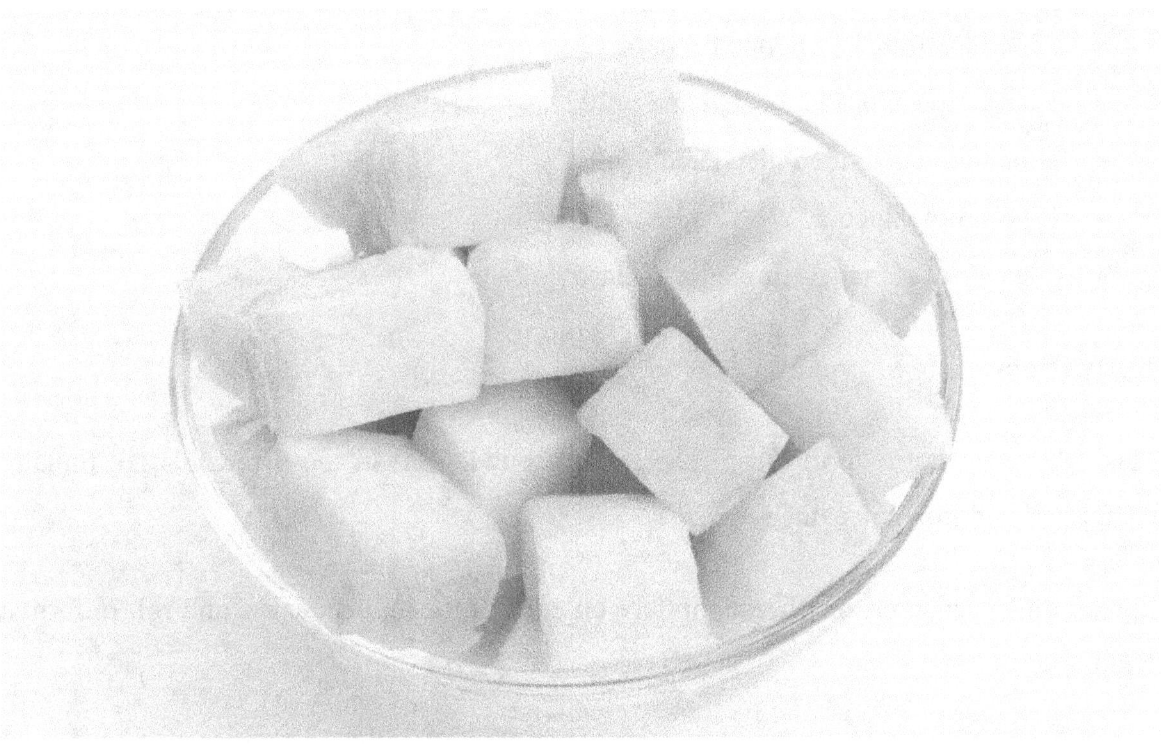

This refreshing recipe combines ripe avocados and sweet mango chunks, nestled within crisp lettuce leaves. A harmonious fusion of textures and tastes, it's a guilt-free delight that satisfies your cravings.

Cooking time: 10 minutes

Servings: 2

Ingredients:

- 1 medium mango, diced
- 1 medium tomato, chopped
- 1 large ripe avocado, peeled and pitted
- 1 medium cucumber, diced and peeled
- 1 Tbsp lime juice
- 6 leaves of romaine lettuce (or collard green)

Instructions:

Mash the avocado to form cream cheese in a bowl. Add in the diced mango, tomato, cucumber, and lime juice, then mix.

Spread the avocado cream cheese mixture on each of the lettuce leaves and roll to form a wrap.

Serve and enjoy!

50. Sweet Honey-Almond Granola

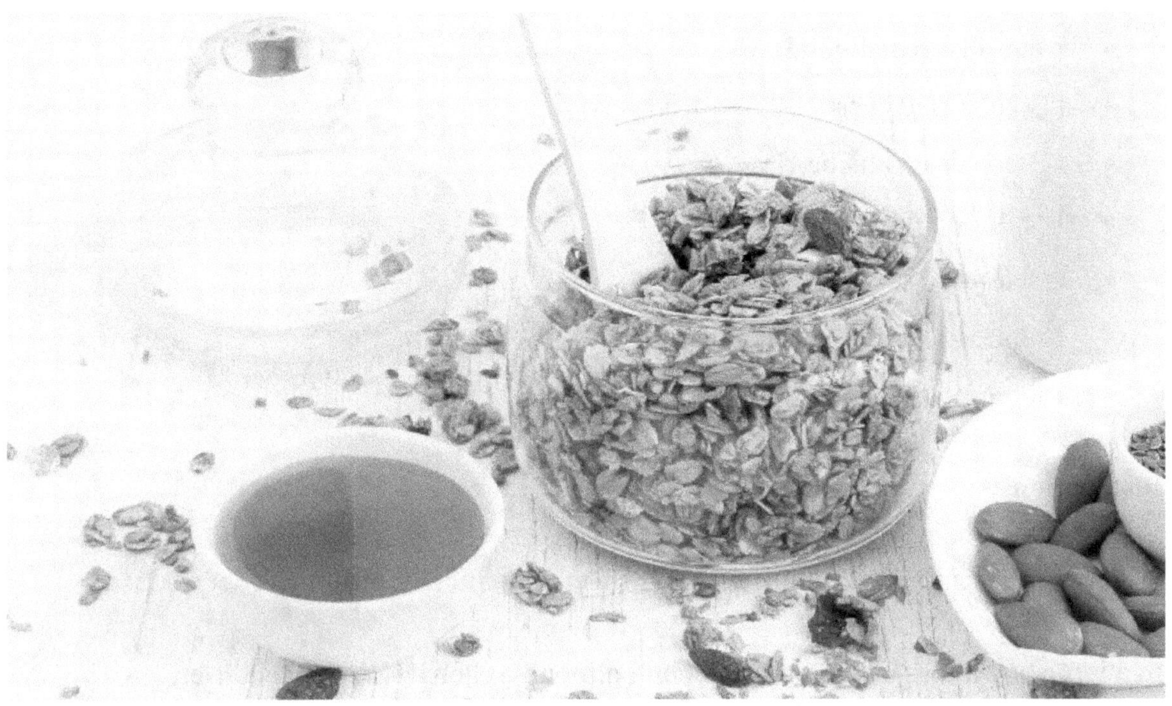

Rich in fiber, this recipe aids digestion and keeps you full. Almonds provide protein, while honey adds natural sweetness. Antioxidants in almonds combat free radicals, promoting skin health.

Cooking time: 15 minutes

Servings: 4

Ingredients:

- 1 cup unsweetened coconut flakes
- 1 cup slivered almonds
- 1/3 cup dried cherries
- 1/3 cup dried blueberries
- 1 teaspoon ground cinnamon
- ½ teaspoon salt
- 1 tablespoon melted coconut oil
- 1 tablespoon honey

Instructions:

Preheat the oven to 300°F. Line a baking sheet with aluminum foil and set aside.

In a large bowl, toss together the coconut, almonds, cherries, and blueberries.

Stir in the cinnamon and salt, mixing well.

Stir in the melted coconut oil and honey, stirring well until all ingredients are coated. Spread the granola mixture on the prepared baking sheet.

Bake for 15 minutes, stirring once halfway through the baking time. Be careful not to overcook. Let cool completely before storing in an airtight container for up to 7 days.

Conclusion

Thank you for reaching the end of this book. I hope this culinary exploration has provided you with valuable insights and practical tools to enhance your well-being.

As you savor the flavors of these thyroid-friendly dishes, remember that your journey to thyroid health is an ongoing process. Embrace it with patience and diligence, making mindful choices to fuel your body with the nutrients it needs. Use this cookbook as a compass to guide you through your culinary adventures, adapting the recipes to your taste preferences and dietary requirements.

Thank You

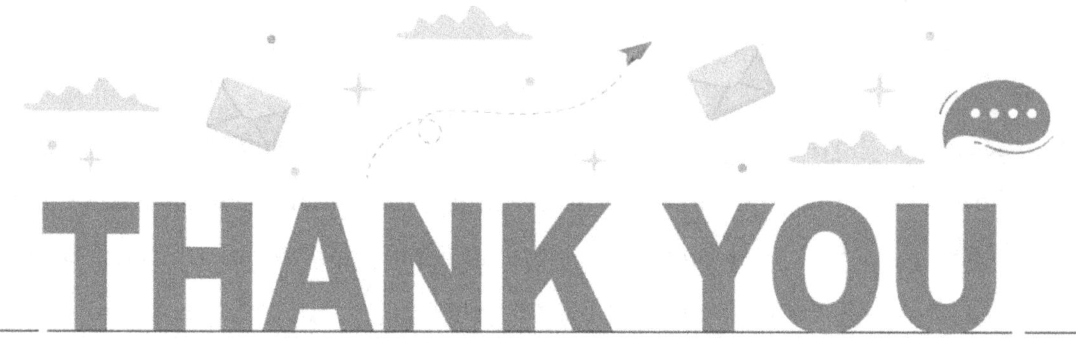

The gratitude I feel for your purchase of my book cannot be expressed in words. Each sale shows me that individuals are benefiting from my experiences and knowledge. Becoming a writer was a decision I made because it allows me to share my skills and expertise with others.

Out of the numerous books available, you chose mine, which is extremely special to me. I have no doubt that the information presented in the book will be useful and informative for you.

Please remember to leave feedback once you've finished reading the book. Every piece of feedback, no matter how small, is invaluable to me in creating even better books. I listen carefully to my readers and take their suggestions into account when developing new content. Your honest feedback will be incorporated into my next books.

Thank you once again for your support.

Alain Duke